The Washington Manual® Internship Survival Guide

Third Edition

Executive Editor

Thomas M. De Fer, MD
Former Barnes-Jewish Hospital Internal Medicine Resident
Associate Professor of Internal Medicine
Washington University School of Medicine
St. Louis, Missouri

Written and Edited by
Bryan A. Faller, MD
Former Barnes-Jewish Hospital Internal Medicine Resident
Instructor of Medicine
Washington University School of Medicine
St. Louis, Missouri

Hemal Gada, MD
Senior Internal Medicine Resident
Barnes-Jewish Hospital
Washington University School of Medicine
St. Louis, Missouri

Sam J. Lubner, MD
Former Barnes-Jewish Hospital Internal Medicine Resident
Instructor of Medicine
Washington University School of Medicine
St. Louis, Missouri

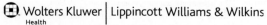

Wolters Kluwer | Lippincott Williams & Wilkins
Health
Philadelphia · Baltimore · New York · London
Buenos Aires · Hong Kong · Sydney · Tokyo

Acquisitions Editor: Ave McCracken
Managing Editor: Michelle LaPlante
Project Manager: Jennifer Harper
Manufacturing Coordinator: Kathleen Brown
Marketing Manager: Kimberly Schonberger
Design Coordinator: Steve Druding
Production Services: International Typesetting and Composition

© **2008 by Department of Medicine, Washington University School of Medicine**
530 Walnut Street
Philadelphia, PA 19106 USA
LWW.com

Second edition, © 2006 Lippincott Williams & Wilkins
First edition, © 2001 Lippincott Williams & Wilkins

Library of Congress Cataloging-in-Publication Data
The Washington manual internship survival guide/executive editor, Thomas
M. De Fer ; written and edited by Bryan A. Faller, Hemal Gada, Sam J.
Lubner.—3rd ed.
  p. ; cm.
  Includes index.
  ISBN 978-0-7817-9360-5
  1. Internal medicine—Handbooks, manuals, etc.   2. Interns
(Medicine)—Handbooks, manuals, etc.   I. DeFer, Thomas M.   II. Faller, Bryan A.
III. Gada, Hemal.   IV. Lubner, Sam J.   V. Washington University (Saint
Louis, Mo.)
  [DNLM: 1. Internal Medicine—Handbooks.   2. Internship and Residency—
Handbooks.   WB 39 W317 2008]
  RC55.L56 2009
  616—dc22   2008000012

To purchase additional copies of this book, call our customer service department at (800) 638-3030
or fax orders to (301) 223-2320. International customers should call (301) 223-2300.

Visit Lippincott Williams & Wilkins on the Internet: at LWW.com. Lippincott Williams & Wilkins
customer service representatives are available from 8:30 am to 6 pm, EST.

10 9 8 7 6 5 4 3 2 1

The Washington Manual® Internship Survival Guide

Third Edition

Preface

This is the third edition of the highly successful, pocket-sized companion "survival guide" written and edited by former Washington University residents. It is meant to be complementary to the *Washington Manual® of Medical Therapeutics* and the *Washington Manual® of Outpatient Internal Medicine* (formerly *Washington Manual® of Ambulatory Medicine*) and to provide concise and practical information for those learning the basics of practicing clinical medicine. It is written assuming knowledge of basic pathophysiology and data interpretation. The target audience is primarily those beginning their internship, but this guide may be useful for medical students, residents, and anyone else on the front lines of patient care.

The third edition has been updated to be consistent with the most current medical practices. The pace of inpatient medicine stresses efficiency and time management, especially in our work-hour regulated environment. In keeping with the purpose of a pocket book, a deliberate attempt was made to keep the format succinct so that common work-ups, cross-cover calls, procedures, and other practical information would always be in a rapidly accessible format. There are also essential sections about "what not to miss" and "when to call for help" for common clinical scenarios. It is written assuming that a standard textbook of internal medicine, the *Washington Manuals®*, a *Sanford Guide*, *Physicians Desk Reference*, and internet access (as well as your resident) are available nearby for reference. Furthermore, we have included a rapid-access, pocket-sized card detailing procedural skills and techniques. This card is detachable, and can travel with you through the course of your residency and beyond.

B.A.F.
H.G.
S.J.L.

Contributing Authors

These authors were all residents or faculty at Washington University at the time of their contributions. Some authors have since moved on to other positions.

Dermatology:

Erica Rogers, MD
Dermatology Resident
Barnes-Jewish Hospital
St. Louis, Missouri

Susan Bayliss, MD
Professor of Dermatology
Washington University School
of Medicine
St. Louis, Missouri
Faculty Advisor

Medical Consultation:

Geoffrey Cislo, MD
Assistant Professor of Medicine
Washington University School
of Medicine
St. Louis, Missouri

Neurology:

Robert Gardner, MD
Neurology Resident
Barnes-Jewish Hospital
St. Louis, Missouri

Richard Sohn, MD
Associate Professor of Neurology
Washington University School
of Medicine
St. Louis, Missouri
Faculty Advisor

Obstetrics and Gynecology:

Andrea Hagemann, MD
Obstetrics and Gynecology
Resident
Barnes-Jewish Hospital
St. Louis, Missouri

Gladys Tse, MD
Assistant Professor of Obstetrics
and Gynecology
Washington University School
of Medicine
St. Louis, Missouri
Faculty Advisor

Ophthalmology:

Matthew Council, MD
Ophthalmology Resident
Barnes-Jewish Hospital
St. Louis, Missouri

Morton Smith, MD
Professor Emeritus of
Ophthalmology
Washington University School
of Medicine
St. Louis, Missouri
Faculty Advisor

Otolaryngology:

Nathan Page, MD
Otolaryngology Resident
Barnes-Jewish Hospital
St. Louis, Missouri

Ravindra Uppaluri, MD, PhD
Assistant Professor of
Otolaryngology
Washington University School
of Medicine
St. Louis, Missouri
Faculty Advisor

Psychiatry:

Nicholas Nguyen, MD
Psychiatry Resident
Barnes-Jewish Hospital
St. Louis, Missouri

Mehmet Dokucu, MD, PhD
Assistant Professor of Psychiatry
Washington University
School of Medicine
St. Louis, Missouri
Faculty Advisor

Radiology:

Meghan Lubner, MD
Radiology Resident
Mallinckrodt Institute of Radiology
Barnes-Jewish Hospital
St. Louis, Missouri

Christine Menias, MD
Assistant Professor of Radiology
Mallinckrodt Institute of Radiology
Washington University School
of Medicine
St. Louis, Missouri
Faculty Advisor

General Surgery:

Elbert Kuo, MD
General Surgery Resident
Barnes-Jewish Hospital
St. Louis, Missouri

Bryan Meyers, MD, MPH
Associate Professor of
Cardiothoracic Surgery
Washington University School
of Medicine
St. Louis, Missouri
Faculty Advisor

Orthopedic Surgery:

David Gerlach, MD
Orthopedic Surgery Resident
Barnes-Jewish Hospital
St. Louis, Missouri

Martin Boyer, MD
Associate Professor of
Orthopedic Surgery
Washington University School
of Medicine
St. Louis, Missouri
Faculty Advisor

Acknowledgments

We wish to thank the following members of the internal medicine residency program at Washington University for their thoughtful comments and suggestions that have made our guide immeasurably better: Suzanne Anderson, MD, Victoria Shekhtman, MD, and Vladimir Kushnir, MD.

We wish to thank Melvin Blanchard, MD, and Kenneth Polonsky, MD, whose leadership and support have been instrumental to the continued success of this book. We appreciate the continued support of Thomas De Fer, MD, and Katherine Henderson, MD, in their coordination of our efforts. From Wolters-Kluwer Health/ Lippincott-Williams & Wilkins, we are indebted to Ave McCracken, Katie Sharp, Michelle LaPlante, and Kimberly Schonberger.

Contents

Abbreviations List

AAA	abdominal aortic aneurysm	JVP	jugular venous pressure
AMA	against medical advice	LBBB	left bundle branch block
AP	anteroposterior	LMWH	low-molecular-weight heparin
APC	atrial premature contraction	LP	lumbar puncture
ARF	acute renal failure	LVH	left ventricular hypertrophy
ATN	acute tubular necrosis	NS	normal saline
AVNRT	AV nodal reentrant tachycardia	NSAID	nonsteroidal anti-inflammatory drug
AVRT	atrioventricular reciprocating tachycardia	NSR	normal sinus rhythm
		PA	posteroanterior
BBB	bundle branch block	PE	physical examination
BP	bullous pemphigoid	PICC	peripherally inserted central catheter
CAD	coronary artery disease		
CHF	congestive heart failure	PID	pelvic inflammatory disease
COPD	chronic obstructive pulmonary disease	PUD	peptic ulcer disease
CPAP	continuous positive airway pressure	PV	pemphigus vulgaris
		PVC	premature ventricular contraction
CXR	chest x-ray		
D/C	discharge	RR	respiratory rate
DKA	diabetic ketoacidosis	RTA	renal tubular acidosis
ECF	extracellular fluid	SBO	small bowel obstruction
FFP	fresh frozen plasma		
GERD	gastroesophageal reflux disease	SBP	systolic BP
		SJS	Stevens-Johnson syndrome
GN	glomerulonephritis		
H&P	history and physical examination	SOB	shortness of breath
		T	temperature
β-hCG	human chorionic gonadotropin-β	TDP	torsades de pointes
		TIA	transient ischemic attack
Hct	hematocrit		
HEENT	head, eyes, ears, nose, and throat	TSH	thyroid-stimulating hormone
HTN	hypertension	TSS	toxic shock syndrome
I/O	input/output	UTI	urinary tract infection
JPCs	junctional premature contractions	VPC	ventricular premature contraction

AAA	abdominal aortic aneurysm
AMA	against medical advice
AP	anteroposterior
APC	atrial premature contraction
ARF	acute renal failure
ATN	acute tubular necrosis
AVNRT	AV nodal reentrant tachycardia
AVRT	atrioventricular reentry tachycardia
BBB	bundle branch block
BP	Bullous pemphigoid
CAD	coronary artery disease
CHF	congestive heart failure
COPD	chronic obstructive pulmonary disease
CPAP	continuous positive airway pressure
CXR	chest x-ray
D/C	discharge
DKA	diabetic ketoacidosis
ECF	extracellular fluid
FFP	fresh frozen plasma
GERD	gastroesophageal reflux disease
GN	glomerulonephritis
H&P	history and physical examination
B-hCG	human chorionic gonadotrophin-B
Hct	hematocrit
HEENT	head, eyes, ears, nose, and throat
HTN	hypertension
I/O	intake/output
3PCs	paroxismal premature contractions

JVP	jugular venous pressure
LBBB	left bundle branch block
LMWH	low-molecular-weight heparin
LP	lumbar puncture
LVH	left ventricular hypertrophy
NS	normal saline
NSAID	nonsteroidal anti-inflammatory drug
NSR	normal sinus rhythm
PA	posteroanterior
PE	physical examination
PICC	peripherally inserted central catheter
PID	pelvic inflammatory diseases
PUD	peptic ulcer disease
PV	pemphigus vulgaris
PVC	premature ventricular contraction
RR	respiratory rate
RTA	renal tubular acidosis
SBO	small bowel obstruction
SBP	systolic BP
SJS	Stevens-Johnson syndrome
SOB	shortness of breath
T	temperature
TDP	torsades de pointes
TIA	transient ischemic attack
TSH	thyroid-stimulating hormone
TSS	toxic shock syndrome
UTI	urinary tract infection
VPC	ventricular premature contraction

Keys to Survival

. . . Or how not *to get voted off of the island . . .*

1. Don't panic.
2. Take care of your patients. You are finally using your education and training.
3. Be kind to the nurses and other ancillary staff. They can make your life much better . . . or much worse.
4. Sleep when you can.
5. Remember to eat.
6. Wear comfortable shoes.
7. Call your significant other when on-call.
8. Verify everything (labs, x-rays, ECGs, etc.) yourself.
9. Ask questions and ask for help. Believe it or not, you are not expected to know everything.
10. Call for consultations on your patients early in the day and have a specific question you want answered from the consultant. This is always appreciated.
11. Start thinking about discharge/disposition planning from day 1.
12. Dictate discharge summaries the day the patient leaves.
13. When generating a differential diagnosis, look for an etiology in VITAMIN E: *V*ascular, *I*nfection/*I*nflammatory, *T*rauma, *A*cquired/*A*utoimmune, *M*etabolic/*M*edications, *I*nherited/*I*atrogenic/*I*diopathic, *N*eoplastic, *E*nvironmental.
14. Work hard, stay enthusiastic, and maintain interest!

ACLS Algorithms

. . . First, take a deep breath. Second, take your own pulse. Now you can begin worrying about the patient . . .

2

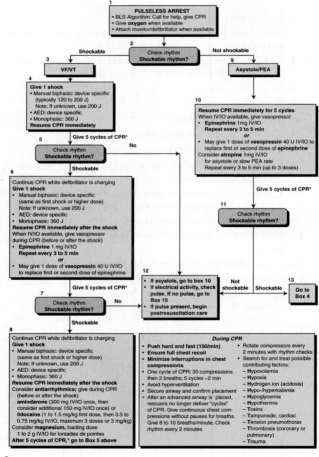

◄—————

Figure 2-1 Advanced Cardiac Life Support Pulseless Arrest algorithm. (From American Heart Association in collaboration with the International Liaison Committee on Resuscitation. Guidelines 2005 for cardiopulmonary resuscitation and emergency cardiovascular care. Part 7.2: Management of cardiac arrest. *Circulation* 2005;112[24 Suppl]:IV59, with permission.)

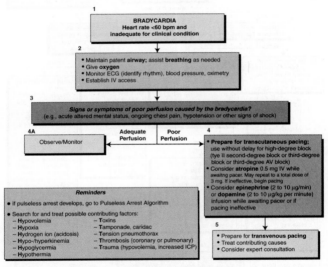

Figure 2-2 Bradycardia algorithm. AV, atrioventricular; bpm, beats per minute; ECG, electrocardiogram; IV, intravenous. (From American Heart Association in collaboration with the International Liaison Committee on Resuscitation. Guidelines 2005 for cardiopulmonary resuscitation and emergency cardiovascular care. Part 7.2: Management of symptomatic bradycardia and tachycardia. *Circulation* 2005;112[24 Supp]:IV68, with permission.)

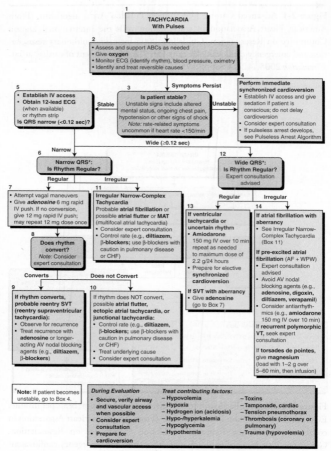

Figure 2-3 Advanced Cardiac Life Support Tachycardia algorithm. (From American Heart Association in collaboration with the International Liaison Committee on Resuscitation. Guidelines 2005 for cardiopulmonary resuscitation and emergency cardiovascular care. Part 7.2: Management of symptomatic bradycardia and tachycardia. *Circulation* 2005;112[24 Suppl]:IV70, with permission.)

Accumulating Your War Chest

3

. . . The best defense is a good offense . . .

BOOKS AND TOOLS TO CARRY WITH YOU

Most house officers carry a compact general manual of internal medicine in their pocket. Many of them are now available in a PDA-supported format. Any of the following are useful and practical:

- Cooper D, Krainik A, Lubner S, Reno H, eds. *The Washington Manual of Medical Therapeutics,* 32nd ed. Lippincott Williams & Wilkins, 2007.
- Nilsson K, Piccini JP, *The Osler Medical Handbook.* Elsevier, 2006.
- Ferri FF, ed. *Practical Guide to the Care of the Medical Patient,* 7th ed. Mosby, 2006.
- Gomella LG, Haist SA. *Clinician's Pocket Reference,* 11th ed. McGraw-Hill Medical, 2006.
- Sabatine, M. *Pocket Medicine.* Lippincott Williams & Wilkins, 2007.
- Dubin D, ed. *Rapid Interpretation of EKG's,* 6th ed. Cover Publishing Company, 2000. (Okay, so it's not likely that you're going to carry this around with you, but it's a great resource to keep in your locker or backpack.)

Other small pocket guides you don't want to be without:

- *Tarascon Pocket Pharmacopoeia.* Tarascon Publishing. Updated yearly.
- Winshall J, Lederman R. *Tarascon Internal Medicine and Critical Care Pocketbook,* 4th ed. Tarascon Publishing, 2006.
- Gilbert DN, Moellering RC, Ellopoulos GM, Sande MA, eds. The Sanford Guide to *Antimicrobial Therapy.* Antimicrobial Therapy Inc. Updated yearly.

Other things to carry with you:

- A good stethoscope
- Reflex hammer

- Guaiac developer and stool cards
- Penlight
- ECG calipers
- Ophthalmoscope/otoscope (yes, you still need this; make sure it's charged for your call and leave it in your locker)
- ABG kit
- Alcohol wipes
- Notecards for patient information

HANDHELD COMPUTER RESOURCES

. . . All in the palm of your hand . . .

Drug References

ePocrates	www.epocrates.com	Free (basic program)/$
Tarascon Pocket Pharmacopoeia	www.tarascon.com	$

Calculators

Many of these programs are embedded in other PDA programs like ePocrates; if you want them individually, here are some links:

MedCalc	www.med-ia.ch/medcalc	Free
ABGPro	www.stacworks.com	Free
Archimedes	www.skyscape.com	Free
ICU Math	www.freewarepalm.com/medical/icumath.shtml	Free

Data Tracking

Patient Keeper	www.patientkeeper.com	$
Patient Tracker	www.handheldmed.com	$

Other References

The Sanford Guide to Antimicrobial Therapy	www.sanfordguide.com	$
Hopkins Antibiotic Guide	www.hopkins-abxguide.org	Free

STATcoder (several guidelines/ calculators)	www.statcoder.com	Free
Journal to Go (journal abstracts and news stories)	www.journaltogo.com	Free
Skyscape (PDA versions of books like the *Washington Manual* and *Harrison's*)	www.Skyscape.com	$

INTERNET RESOURCES

. . . Unfortunately, sleep is not downloadable at this time . . .

General Sites

UpToDate	www.uptodate.com	$
Medscape	www.medscape.com	
eMedicine	www.emedicine.com	
National Guidelines Clearinghouse	www.guideline.gov	
MD Consult	www.mdconsult.com	$
American College of Physicians	www.acponline.org	

Cardiovascular Disease

| National Heart, Lung, and Blood Institute | www.nhlbi.nih.gov |
| American College of Cardiology | www.acc.org |

Cerebrovascular Disease and Stroke

National Institute of Neurological Diseases	www.ninds.nih.gov
National Stroke Association	www.stroke.org
Washington University	www.strokecenter .org

Pulmonary Diseases and Allergy

| American College of Chest Physicians | www.chestnet.org |

Endocrine and Diabetes

National Institute of Diabetes and Digestive and Kidney Diseases	www.niddk.nih.gov
American Diabetes Association	www.diabetes.org
The Endocrine Society	www.endo-society.org
American Thyroid Association	www.thyroid.org

Rheumatology

National Institute of Arthritis and Musculoskeletal and Skin Diseases	www.niams.nih.gov
American College of Rheumatology	www.rheumatology.org

Nephrology

National Institute of Diabetes and Digestive and Kidney Diseases	www.niddk.nih.gov
RenalNet-Kidney Information Clearinghouse	www.renalnet.org
National Kidney Foundation	www.kidney.org

Oncology

National Cancer Institute	www.cancer.gov
National Comprehensive Cancer Network	www.nccn.org

Orthopaedic Surgery

American Association of Orthopaedic Surgeons	www.orthoinfo.aaos.org

Gastroenterology

American Gastroenterological Association	www.gastro.org
American College of Gastroenterology	www.acg.gi.org

Infectious Disease/HIV

University of California at San Francisco—HIV site	hivinsite.ucsf.edu
Centers for Disease Control and Prevention	www.cdc.gov
National Institute of Allergy and Infectious Diseases	www.niaid.nih.gov
World Health Organization	www.who.int

Geriatrics, Aging, Osteoporosis

Alzheimer's Disease Education and Referral Center	www.alzheimers.org
Administration on Aging	www.aoa.dhhs.gov

Complementary and Alternative Medicine

National Center for Complementary and Alternative Medicine	nccam.nih.gov
Medline Plus	www.nlm.nih.gov/medlineplus/herbalmedicine.html

Online Journals (subscriptions may be required)

Annals of Internal Medicine	www.annals.org
British Medical Journal	www.bmj.com
Journal of the American Medical Association	www.jama.ama-assn.org
The Lancet	www.thelancet.com
New England Journal of Medicine	www.nejm.org

INTERNET RESOURCES FOR EVIDENCE-BASED MEDICINE

The library at your institution is a great place to start for EBM searches. Many of them offer web-based proxy servers to their e-journal collections, as well as search engines like PubMed or Ovid.

The Cochrane Database of Systematic Reviews

http://thecochranelibrary.net
Reviews, analyzes, and synthesizes the best clinical trials by topics.
Multi-directional links MEDLINE, EBM, and EUCLID full-text. Subscription required.

PubMed

www.ncbi.nlm.nih.gov/entrez/
Maintained by the National Library of Medicine
Allows a user-friendly approach to medical literature with built-in search filters. Free.

ACP Journal Club

www.acpjc.org
Evidence-based medicine reviews of journal articles. Subscription required.

Useful Formulas

4

. . . Corrected Sleep Equation . . .

$$\text{Sleep (hours)} = \frac{(\text{Discharges} + \text{Transfers})/}{(\text{Admissions} + \text{Cross-Cover})^2} \times \#\text{Interns}$$

A-a O$_2$ GRADIENT

A-a gradient = $PAO_2 - PaO_2$; $PAO_2 = (FiO_2 \times 713) - PaCO_2/0.8$
(all units in mmHg)

- Estimate for upper limit of normal in room air (in mmHg) by age = (Age/4 + 4)

Causes of Increased A-a Gradient

- $\dot{V}/\dot{Q}$ mismatch
- Intrapulmonary right-to-left shunt
- Intracardiac right-to-left shunt
- Impaired diffusion (room air only)

ANION GAP (SERUM)

$AG = [Na^+] - ([Cl^-] + [HCO^-_3])$
([Na$^+$], [Cl$^-$], HCO$^-_3$] in meq/L)
Normal = 8–12 mEq/L
See Acid-Base section in Chapter 16 for differential diagnosis.

ANION GAP (URINE)

$UAG = (U[Na^+] + U[K^+]) - U[Cl^-]$
(U[Na$^+$], U[K$^+$], U[Cl$^-$] in meq/L)

- Normal = slightly positive

- UAG is **negative** in diarrhea-induced nongap metabolic acidosis (**enhanced** urinary NH_4 excretion).
- UAG is **positive** in distal RTA–induced nongap metabolic acidosis (**impaired** urinary NH_4 excretion).

BODY MASS INDEX

$BMI = Wt(kg)/(Ht(m))^2$

- Interpretation: <18.5 = underweight; 18.5–24.9 = normal weight; 25–29.9 = overweight; >30 = obese.

CREATININE CLEARANCE

Estimated (Cockcroft–Gault Formula):
$CrCl = (140 - age) \times weight/Cr \times 72$
Multiply by 0.85 for women.
(*Weight in kg, Cr in mg/dL*)

Measured:
$CrCl = U[Cr] \times U_{volume}/P[Cr] \times time$
(*Cr in mg/dL, volume in mL, and time in min*)
Normal CrCl >100 mL/min

CORRECTED SERUM CALCIUM

Corrected serum Ca = measured $[Ca^{+2}]$ + $[0.8 \times (4.0 - measured\ albumin)]$
        (*$[Ca^{+2}]$ in mg/dL, albumin in g/day*)

CORRECTED SERUM SODIUM

Corrected serum Na = measured $[Na^+]$ + $[0.016 \times (measured\ [glucose] - 100)]$
        (*$[Na^+]$ in meq/L, [glucose] in mg/dL*)

FRACTIONAL EXCRETION OF SODIUM

$$FENa = U[Na^+] \times P[Cr]/P[Na^+] \times U[Cr] \times 100$$

(U[Na$^+$] and P[Na$^+$] in meq/L; U[Cr] and P[Cr] in mg/dL)

FENa <1% in prerenal states, early ATN, contrast or heme pigment nephropathy, and acute glomerulonephritis; not valid when diuretics have been given.

FRACTIONAL EXCRETION OF UREA

$$FEurea = (U[urea] \times P[Cr]/BUN \times U[Cr]) \times 100$$

(All units in mg/dL)

FEurea <35% in prerenal states; not affected by diuretics.

MEAN ARTERIAL PRESSURE

$$MAP = SBP + (2 \times DBP)/3$$

OSMOLALITY (SERUM, ESTIMATED)

Calculated serum osm =

$$(2 \times [Na+]) + [glucose]/18 + [BUN]/2.8.$$

([Na$^+$] in meq/L; [glucose] and [BUN] in mg/dL)

OSMOLAL GAP

Osmolal gap = measured S_{osm} − calculated S_{osm}

Causes of Increased Osmolal Gap

Decreased serum water, hyperproteinemia, hypertriglyceridemia, and presence of unmeasured osmoles (sorbitol, glycerol, mannitol, ethanol, isopropyl alcohol, acetone, ethyl ether, methanol, and ethylene glycol).

RETICULOCYTE INDEX

Reticulocyte index = Observed reticulocyte count × (Measured Hct %/ 45 %)/ Maturation Index

- Maturation index = 1 + (0.5 × (45-Hct)10)
- Good marrow response = 3.0–6.0; Borderline response = 2.0–3.0; Inadequate response = <2.0

MEDICAL EPIDEMIOLOGY

- **Sensitivity:** The percentage of patients with the target disorder who have a positive result (A/[A + C]). The greater the sensitivity, the more likely the test will detect patients with the disease. High sensitivity tests are useful clinically to rule OUT a disease (SnOUT) (i.e., a negative test result would virtually exclude the possibility of the disease) (Table 4-1).
- **Specificity:** The percentage of patients without the target disorder who have a negative test result (D/[B + D]). Very specific tests are used to confirm or rule IN the presence of disease (SpIN).
- **Positive predictive value (PPV):** The percentage of persons with positive test results who actually have the disease (A/[A + B]).
- **Negative predictive value (NPV):** The percentage of persons with negative test results in which the disease is absent (D/[C + D]).
- **Number needed to treat (NNT):** The number of patients who need to be treated to achieve one additional favorable outcome; calculated as 1/absolute risk reduction (ARR), rounded up to the nearest whole number.
- **Number needed to harm (NNH):** The number of patients who, if they received the experimental treatment, would lead to one additional person being harmed compared with patients who receive the control treatment; calculated as 1/absolute risk increase (ARI).

TABLE 4-1   MEDICAL EPIDEMIOLOGY

Test Result	Disease	No Disease		
Positive	Truepositive (A)	False positive (B)	All with positive test (A+B)	Positive predictive value (PPV) = $\dfrac{\text{True positives}}{\text{All with positive test}}$ (A/[A + B])
Negative	False negative (C)	True negative (D)	All with negative test (C + D)	Negative predictive value (NPV) = $\dfrac{\text{True negatives}}{\text{All with negative test}}$ (C/[C + D])
	All patients who have disease (A + C)	All patients without disease (B + D)		
	Sensitivity = (A/[A + C])	Specificity = (D/[B + D])		

Triage

BEFORE ACCEPTING ADMISSIONS

. . . Do ask, do tell . . .

1. Obtain vital stats: name, date of birth, medical record number, current location, and attending physician.
2. Why does the patient need to be admitted?
3. Is the patient competent, and does he or she want to be admitted?
4. What are the patient's chief complaints, comorbidities, relevant past medical history, and brief current history?
5. When was the last previous admission? Obtain old medical records (inpatient and outpatient). If the patient is coming in transfer, be sure to acquire all radiographs and lab results.
6. Obtain most recent vital signs, pertinent examination including mental status, key lab data, CXR, ECG, and code status. Review as many lab results and films in the ED as you can.
7. Confirm IV access.
8. Inquire about major interventions performed, medications given, and consultations pending.
9. What follow-up is necessary (i.e., lab tests that are pending, consults that need to be called, blood transfusions, antibiotics)?
10. Find out who the primary MD is and if this person has been notified.
11. Do family members need to be called?

OTHER IMPORTANT QUESTIONS TO CONSIDER

. . . Location, location, location . . .

• Is this an appropriate admission for your service (i.e., is there something you can do for the patient that no one else can do? Does a different service make more sense?)?

- Can this patient be managed as an outpatient? If yes, social services may need to be involved. In addition, arranging follow-up is crucial.
- Is the patient stable enough for the floor? Are any more treatments needed before transfer to the floor (i.e., nebulizer treatments, etc.)?
- Can your staff adequately handle this patient?
- What specific interventions does this patient need that other institutions cannot provide (in the case of a hospital-to-hospital transfer)?

Obtain collateral information from family, nursing homes, or other caregivers. Always collect and hold on to important phone contacts.

Cross-Coverage

. . . Who? What? Wait, let me get my sign-out . . .

GENERAL POINTS

1. For the first few months of residency, when you are called about a patient, it is a good idea to go see the patient, reference the chart, and assess the situation. Do this until you feel comfortable deciding what situations can be adequately handled over the telephone with the nurses and the support staff.

2. Always go see the patient if you have any doubt or concern. The patient is always your number one priority.

3. If you do go see a patient, always write an event note (this can be brief, depending on the situation). Things to document include:

   A. Reason you were called to see patient (e.g., CTSP for chest pain).

   B. Assessment of situation on arrival including general appearance, vitals, pertinent physical examination, pertinent laboratory and imaging data.

   C. Interventions.

   D. Outcome.

REASONS YOU MUST GO SEE A PATIENT

. . . Drop everything and go now. Godspeed . . .

1. Any major changes in clinical status.
   - Altered mental status or other changes in neurologic state.
   - Dyspnea.
   - Chest pain.
   - Severe abdominal pain.
   - Seizures.

- Uncontrolled bleeding (hemoptysis, hematemesis, lower GI bleed, hematuria, vaginal bleeding).
- Uncontrolled vomiting.
- Severe headache.
- New onset of pain.
- Falls.

2. Any major changes in vital signs.
   - Oxygen desaturation.
   - Hypotension.
   - Arrhythmias (tachyarrhythmias and bradyarrhythmias).
   - Fever associated with changes in mental status, changes in other vital signs.

THINGS TO CONSIDER ASKING FOR BEFORE ARRIVAL AT BEDSIDE

. . . Delegate before it's too late . . .

1. In situations in which the patient is becoming unstable or you are at all unsure, page the resident immediately!
2. Full set of vitals.
3. Hospital chart at bedside.
4. IV access.
5. Oxygen (nasal cannula, face mask), respiratory therapist.
6. Cardiac monitor, ECG.
7. Crash/code cart.
8. Chest x-ray.
9. ABG kits.
10. Blood cultures, if febrile.
11. Basic lab results.
12. Restraints.

THINGS THAT CAN WAIT

. . . Passing back the pain . . .

1. Talking to family members; unless urgent, this can usually be handled by the primary team.

2. Major adjustments in medication regimen in a stable patient (i.e., diabetic medicines, antihypertensive medicines, antibiotics).

3. Consultations in nonemergent, stable situations (i.e., GI consult in patient with Hemoccult-positive brown stool, stable hematocrit, stable vital signs).

4. Addressing code status in a stable patient.

APPROPRIATE TRANSFER OF PATIENTS TO THE INTENSIVE CARE UNIT

. . . Passing on the pain . . .

1. Determine which unit is most appropriate for management of the patient.
2. Speak to the resident who will be accepting the patient to inform him or her of the situation.
3. Have the nursing staff give report to the staff in the unit.
4. Every patient needs a brief transfer note, including:
    A. When and why you were called to see the patient.
    B. One-line description of patient and his or her comorbidities.
    C. Your assessment of the situation.
    D. Your management of the situation, including diagnostic and therapeutic measures, complications, and outcome. Include code note, if appropriate.
    E. Your assessment and plan at this point with brief differential diagnosis of what could be going on.
    F. Reason for transfer (pressors, arrhythmias, unstable vital signs, closer monitoring, etc.).
    G. Vascular access (femoral line, peripheral IV, etc.).
    H. Code status.
    I. Who has been notified (patient's physician, family members).

Patient and Staff Relations 7

. . . It's like winking in the dark, you know what you're doing, but make sure everyone else does, too . . .

WORKING WITH ANCILLARY STAFF

- Give specific directions and use your judgment, but also give others a chance to make suggestions and solve problems. Effective use of ancillary staff can greatly increase your efficiency.
- A compliment for a job well done goes a long way (others are overworked, too), and you will be remembered when you need help. When someone performs exemplary work, let his or her supervisor know.
- Criticize in private. Constructive feedback may be necessary and welcomed if done in a nonjudgmental manner.
- Regard ancillary staff as fellow members of the patient care team; they are often "bothering" you out of concern for the patient and not to harass you. They have valuable insight that often proves important in patient care.
- Efforts to let team members know the plan can save you phone calls and increase sleep.

REFERRING A PATIENT

- When referring a patient to the ED, another physician, or transferring a patient, always make a courtesy call first.
- Pertinent information includes:
  1. Who you are.
  2. Patient identification information.
  3. Succinct history of the problem.
  4. Supporting lab data.
  5. Suggestions for further evaluation.

6. Likely disposition of the patient.
7. A contact number where you or someone covering for you can be reached for questions or follow-up information.

WORKING WITH DIFFICULT PATIENTS

. . . Having fun yet? . . .

- Be proactive and address potential concerns, expectations, or questions up front. Checking in with the patient at regular intervals builds rapport and can save you from multiple phone calls. Try to minimize waiting time and interruptions during meetings.
- Be as flexible and as accommodating as you can. Recognize that the patient may be tired of repeating his or her history or having a physical examination.
- Letting the patient (and loved ones) know about the management plan should be done at least once a day. Follow up with them on test results and changes in the plan, and let them know if consultants will be coming by.
- If more than one service is involved, designate someone to be the primary source of communication to avoid confusion.
- The patient's "difficult" behavior may stem from lack of control over decision making and the situation or lack of insight into his or her medical condition. Past experiences, things the patient may have seen or read in the media, and fear may also play a role. *Active* listening, acknowledging the patient's point of view, and reassurance can go a long way.
- Acknowledge your own frustration, seek the advice of others when necessary, and always try to do what's best for the patient.

TABLE 7-1 DEALING WITH DIFFICULT PROBLEMS

Problems	Suggestions	Potential Actions
Abuses of the system (i.e., narcotics)	Set boundaries; written contracts are often helpful (be specific in stating the problem and plan).	Notify all members of the team caring for the patient. Document concisely in the chart and include on sign out.
Manipulative patients	See above. Coordinate care through one team member to maintain consistency.	See above.
Violent patients (see Chapter 17, Psychiatry section)	Safety first. Tell others you are seeing the patient. Try to remain calm and neutral. Always stand between the patient and the door. Remove all potentially dangerous items that can be used against you (i.e., stethoscope).	See above. Contact security or law enforcement officials if necessary. Arrange to have security nearby when you see the patient.
Patients who want to leave AMA	First, establish decisional capacity (see Chapter 17, Psychiatry consultation section). Then, listen to the patient's reason(s).	See above. Have patient sign AMA form. Carefully document discussion of risks and benefits in the chart.

22

	Respond in a nondefensive, nonjudgmental manner. Calmly explain the risks and consequences of leaving. Explain the benefits of staying and the importance of completing the diagnostic/treatment plan. Be accommodating if possible. Enlist the help of other team/family members.	Try to arrange discharge medications and follow-up plans. Advise the patient to seek medical attention again if condition worsens. Notify the attending of record of AMA discharge.
Homelessness or return to abusive situations	Social work is a helpful resource.	Refer patients to local shelters or to local shelters/safe havens. Contact proper authorities (i.e., police, Division of Aging, Child and Family Services). Careful, neutral documentation in the medical record.
Refusal of nursing home placement	Social work, family members, and other team members can assist and discuss with patient. Consider rehabilitation as a potential place for referral.	Emphasize that it may be a temporary stay. Try to arrange for close out-patient follow-up, home health services, and other family members to check in and help.

(Continued)

TABLE 7-1	DEALING WITH DIFFICULT PROBLEMS *(continued)*	
Problems	**Suggestions**	**Potential Actions**
High likelihood that patient will abuse substances again	Consider chemical dependency consult.	Ultimately, you may have to respect the patient's wishes. Educate the patient on hazards of substance abuse. Consider inpatient or outpatient follow-up.
Concern for suicide or homicide (see Chapter 17, Psychiatry section)	Consider psychiatry consultation, assess competency.	Document carefully in the chart. Place patient on suicide precautions with sitter. Consider possible transfer to inpatient psychiatric setting.
Financial difficulties	Social workers or case coordinators can be very helpful.	Notify family members and loved ones. Payment and transportation arrangements can be made. Medication samples. Referral to free clinics and resources. Assistance with applying for Medicaid, disability, etc.

TABLE 7-2	POTENTIAL RESOURCES AND OPTIONS
Resources	**Options**
Nursing supervisor or manager	Individual or joint meetings with or without loved ones (useful for any situation below).
Social worker	Initial evaluation for nursing home, rehab, or extended care facility placement.
Case coordinator	Return to nursing home issues; durable medical equipment; insurance disputes and concerns.
	Home health/home infusion/ hospice referrals.
	Transportation issues.
Risk management	For litigious patients/family members, if you have concerns about the case, or if you expect a poor outcome.
Ombudsman or ethics committee	Helpful if there are disputes between physicians or family members.
Family members or loved ones	Proceed cautiously; if there are family members who are in disagreement, try to remain neutral.
Religious resources	For spiritual support and issues related to death and end of life.
A new physician	A new physician may be the best solution if other options have failed.

TABLE 7-3	ADDRESSING END-OF-LIFE ISSUES

Issue	Suggestions
Code status	Explain it in language and terms the patient and family members can understand.
Intubation	
CPR	
Vasopressors	Remain neutral, although it is appropriate to give your opinion, especially if asked.
Cardioversion	
Antibiotics and other medications	Be very specific and clear (i.e., the exact interventions to be done or not to be done) in your discussion and **document clearly in the medical record.**
Nutrition (i.e., G-tubes)	
Phlebotomy	
IV lines	
Withdrawal of support	**Communicate status with other team members.**
Comfort care	
	Give sufficient time to consider the decision, and explain this decision can be changed.
	Be open and available for further discussion and questions.
	If patient is not able to discuss this with you, contact primary physician and family members, power of attorney.

Admissions

Admission

$$\text{Pain Index} = \frac{\text{Patient's age (years)} \times \text{Length of stay (days)}}{\text{Glasgow Coma Scale score}}$$

(Harris index)

GENERAL POINTS

1. When called with a new admission, it is critical to review old records, lab results, and old charts. However, if the patient is accessible, always eyeball the patient first and check vital signs before digging through old records. With that said, old records are invaluable. Most systems have old lab results, discharge summaries, and H & Ps stored as electronic versions; use these extensively, but always confirm with your own eyes and ears.

2. After assessment of the patient and examination, admission orders should be completed as soon as possible. This will help the nursing staff and will enable you to get appropriate lab results in a timely manner. If you need stat labs, always inform the nursing staff directly. It is also helpful to inform the nurses when your orders are complete. Telemetry orders should also be completed as soon as possible if needed.

3. The history and physical examination should be well ingrained by now. It is often helpful to dictate the H & P right after evaluating the patient. If you decide to dictate, you must ensure a signed copy of the dictation makes it into the medical record chart. A short handwritten note of the current admission problems and short assessment should also be entered in the chart while awaiting the dictated H & P. Lab results can be added manually to the dictation as an addendum.

4. If the patient has a private primary care physician, he or she should be notified as soon as possible regarding the admission, and your plan should be communicated to the private physician. Many private physicians or their covering partners like to be notified as soon as possible, regardless of the time of night.

5. In summary, remember the three pearls of an admission:
   - Assess the stability of the patient: *Do this first.*
   - Obtain a good H & P, even if this has already been done by another medical team.
   - Write orders as soon as possible. This makes the nurses and unit clerks happy and allows you to get the lab data you need to finish your evaluation.

ADMISSION ORDERS

Many admission diagnoses have preset clinical pathways and associated order sets (i.e., CHF, asthma). These are often helpful. Also, consider the patient's eligibility for appropriate research studies.

The mnemonic ADC VAANDISML may be useful:

Admit to ward/attending/house officers.

Diagnosis.

Condition.

Vitals: e.g., routine, every shift, every 2 hours. Always include call orders (i.e., call HO for SBP >180 or <90, pulse >130 or <60, RR >30 or <10, T >38.3°C, O2 saturation <92%).

Allergies and reactions.

Activity (ad lib, bedrest with bedside commode, up to chair, etc.).

Nursing (strict I/O, daily weights, guaiac stools, Accuchecks, Foleys, etc.).

Diet (NPO, prudent diabetic, low fat/low cholesterol, renal, low salt, etc.).

IV (IV fluids, heplock).

Special (wound care, consults with social work, dietitian, and PT/OT).

Meds: All medications should include dosage, timing, route, and indications. Don't forget prn meds or you will be called often; if no contraindications, include acetaminophen (Tylenol), bisacodyl (Dulcolax) or docusate (Colace), and aluminum and magnesium hydroxide (Maalox).

Laboratory (don't forget to include a.m. labs).

Don't forget DVT prophylaxis for every patient who is not ambulating and GI prophylaxis for critically ill patients (see below for guidelines)!

DVT PROPHYLAXIS

- Indications: Patients with one or more risk factors and confined to bed; critical care patients.
- Risk factors for DVT: Cardiac dysfunction (heart failure, arrhythmia, MI), malignancy, surgery, trauma (especially orthopedic), previous DVT, obesity, smoking, age >40 years, inflammatory disease (e.g., inflammatory bowel disease, lupus), nephrotic syndrome, pregnancy or postpartum within 1 month, immobility, acquired or genetic thrombophilia, chronic lung disease.
- Contraindications to pharmacologic prophylaxis: heparin-induced thrombocytopenia, active bleeding, preoperative within 12 hours or postoperative within 24 hours, LP or epidural within 24 hours; recent intraocular or intracranial surgery; coagulopathy.
- Recommended regimens (for medical patients):
  - Low-molecular-weight heparins (LMWH): enoxaparin 40 mg subcutaneous q day, dalteparin 5,000 units subcutaneous q day, or fondaparinux 2.5 mg subcutaneous q day. Adjust dosage for CrCl <30 mg/dL.
  - Unfractionated heparin (UFH) 5,000 subcutaneous bid or tid.
  - For patients at high risk of bleeding, consider intermittent pneumatic compression or graduated compression stockings.
- For planned invasive procedures (e.g., pacemaker placement, catheterization, surgery, etc.), hold UFH 8 hours prior to procedure and LMWH 12 hours prior to procedure!

GI PROPHYLAXIS

- Gastric erosions and stress-induced ulcers can form in critically ill patients. However, not every patient needs GI prophylaxis—if patients do not have any of the risk factors listed below, prophylaxis is not necessary, even in the ICU setting! Most patient will *not* need GI prophylaxis.

- Risk factors for stress-induced ulcers: Mechanical ventilation >48 hours, coagulopathy, shock, sepsis, multi-organ system failure, hepatic failure, multiple trauma, burns >35% of total body surface area, organ transplant recipient, head trauma, spinal cord injury, history of peptic ulcer disease or upper GI bleeding, use of anticoagulants or high dose corticosteroids.
- Recommended regimens:
  - H2 blockers: e.g., famotidine 20 mg PO/IV bid or ranitidine 50 mg PO/IV tid.
  - Proton-pump inhibitors: e.g., omeprazole 40 mg PO q day.

ASSESSMENT/PLAN

This is the meat of your note. It is useful to separate this section by problem. The assessment should include a one-line summary of the patient's known medical problems (i.e., HTN, T2DM, CAD) and those under evaluation (i.e., fever, melena). For example, 60 y/o female with a history of hypertension, T2DM presents with new onset chest pain. Include a short differential diagnosis of the current problem.

The plan should be separated by problem. Cover all problems, including stable issues:

1. Chest pain: No ECG changes, chest pain free now, will rule out MI, monitor on telemetry, continue beta blocker, nitrates, ASA, and ACE-I. NPO for stress thallium in AM assuming rules out for MI.

2. Hypertension: Good control on current medical regimen.

3. T2DM: Good control with A1C of 6.5. Continue glucose checks, prudent diabetic diet. Hold PO diabetic meds while NPO. Will use insulin sliding scale while NPO.

4. Fluids/electrolytes/nutrition (F/E/N): Monitor I/O's, urine output.

5. Vascular access: Note patient's sites of IV access.

6. Prophylaxis: Indicate plans for DVT prophylaxis and GI prophylaxis if indicated (see above).

7. Disposition: Note any discharge needs (nursing home placement, home health, home O$_2$, etc.).

8. Code status: Code status should be addressed with every patient admitted regardless of age or disease. Unexpected problems arise too often, and it is better to be prepared.

LABORATORY RESULTS AND ORDERS

It is imperative that orders and lab tests are followed up in a timely manner. You must take personal responsibility to ensure that this is completed.

PATIENT SAFETY ISSUES

Restraints

Restraints may be needed for patients in a variety of situations. Indications for restraints include:

- Protecting patients from harming themselves (e.g., self-extubation, pulling at Foley catheter, pulling at IV lines).
- Protecting staff and/or family from patient violence.
- Facilitating medically necessary procedures.
- Preventing disoriented patients from wandering or falls.

Written orders for restraints must include:

- Type of restraint (e.g., soft limb restraints, mittens).
- Start and end times.
- Frequency of monitoring and reevaluation.

Medical reason for restraint use must be documented in the chart. Patients should be reevaluated at least every 24 hours and orders renewed if necessary. Consider the use of chemical restraints (e.g., benzodiazepines or antipsychotics), bedside sitters, bed alarms, or veil beds instead of physical restraints if possible. Most hospitals have written policies regarding the use of restraints—be sure your orders and documentation comply with hospital policies.

Dangerous Abbreviations for Order Writing

Each hospital may have its own list of unacceptable or dangerous abbreviations, but Table 8.1 shows some of the most common.

TABLE 8-1   DANGEROUS ABBREVIATIONS FOR ORDER WRITING

Abbreviation	Intended Meaning	Misinterpretation/Common Error	Correction
U	Units	Mistaken for the numbers "0" or "4", or "cc"	Write "unit"
IU	International Units	Mistaken for "IV" or the number "10"	Write "International Units"
Q.D. or Q.O.D	Daily or every other day	Mistaken for each other, or QID	Write "daily" Write "every other day"
Trailing zero or lack of leading zero	X.0 mg or .X mg	Decimal point is missing	Write X mg Write 0.X mg
MS, MSO, and MgSO	Morphine sulfate or magnesium sulfate	Confused for one another	Write "morphine sulfate". Write "magnesium sulfate"
μg	Microgram	Mistaken for "mg"	Use "mcg" or "microgram"
AU, AS, AD	Latin abbreviation for both ears, left ear, right ear	Mistaken as the Latin abbreviation "OU" (both eyes); "OS" (left eye); "OD" right eye	Write "both ears"; "left ear" or "right ear"
CC	Cubic centimeter	Misread as "U" (Units)	Use "mL" or "ml"; or write out "cubic centimeters" or "milliliters"
HS	Half strength or Latin abbreviation for bedtime	Confused for either half strength or at bedtime; qHS mistaken for every hour	Write out "half strength" or "at bedtime"
TIW	Three times a week	Misinterpreted as "three times a day" or "twice a week"	Write "three times a week" or specify days (e.g., Q MWF)

From Barnes-Jewish Hospital Department of Pharmacy. St. Louis: Washington University Medical Center, July 2007.

Daily Assessments

9

. . . Same bat time, same bat channel . . .

ROUNDS

. . . Round and round and round . . .

Many programs categorize rounds into prerounds, work rounds, and attending rounds.

Prerounding

Prerounding is primarily an intern's responsibility. Usually allow 30 minutes to an hour before rounds, depending on the number of patients on your service. The exact responsibilities should be worked out individually with your resident. It is often not necessary to physically see all of your patients before work rounds. It is customary to see those patients with an acute problem.

Probably the most important aspects are getting signouts and catching up on the overnight events (i.e., cross-cover problems). However, the following example is a good prerounding plan:

1. Get your signout from the night float or cross-cover team. You need to know of any major events that happened overnight, and this dictates how you will spend your time prerounding.

2. Check vital signs on all your patients. This can often be done on the computers. It is also helpful to check nursing notes on the computer.

3. See the patients. A quick check on your patients (2–3 minutes per patient) allows you to see how they look and if they have developed any new problems overnight. Of course, patients with more acute illness require more time.

4. Check lab results and final results of tests (i.e., CXR, echos, etc.). Check telemetry every day on all your monitored patients.

5. For patients with private physicians, it is often helpful to discuss the plan face-to-face with them in the morning (i.e., try

to catch them on their morning rounds). This saves you time in trying to reach them at their offices or in deciphering their progress notes.

DAILY NOTES AND EVALUATION

Interns are primarily responsible for writing daily notes on each of their patients. The SOAP format is usually used for daily notes.

Subjective: What the patient says or what nursing staff reports. Past 24 hour events.

Objective: Factual information, vitals, PE, lab results, lines, and tubes. Include microbiology results, x-rays, and other studies here. Always check final official readings of tests.

Assessment/Plan: This is the meat of the note. Usually categorized by problem or organ system in the order of importance. Always include fluids/electrolytes/nutrition as a problem as well as code status in every note. Also include the type of IV access the patient has and plan for DVT prophylaxis. The last category or problem should be discharge planning. Include status and goals (e.g., social work placement, home oxygen).

Active medications are often listed in a side column. This exercise can be tedious but ensures that every medication is reviewed daily. Also include the day number for antibiotics and other loading dose medications.

Review the following items daily:

- Do IV lines need to be changed?
- Can IV meds be changed to PO?
- Can you discontinue the Foley?
- Do restraint orders need to be renewed?
- Can you advance the diet and increase the activity of the patient? Is the patient moving his or her bowels? Is there any procedure or test planned that requires that patient to be NPO?
- PT/OT and social work: Are they involved, and should they be? What is the status of discharge planning?
- Are all meds adjusted for renal or hepatic failure?

Daily orders should be consolidated and written as early as possible. Don't forget to order AM labs for the next morning. Every lab test and study ordered needs to be followed up. If a study needs to be done stat or ASAP, you must notify the ward clerk and nurse directly, and consider talking to the radiologist directly. It is often helpful to discuss a brief plan with the patient and the nursing staff. This helps them to be part of the team and also helps move things along.

DISCHARGE PLANNING

D/C planning must be addressed and readdressed constantly. Proper D/C planning prevents large teams and reduces resident irritation. D/C planning should start on admission. Social work should be consulted on admission if D/C needs are anticipated (assisted living, placement, transportation). Scheduled meetings with case coordinators or social workers are often helpful to reassess the situation and provide updates.

SIGNOUTS

Most programs have some variety of night float to help with cross-cover overnight. Succinct but complete signouts include the following items:

- Name of patient, birth date, room number.
- List of active problems and relevant medical history (i.e., ESRD).
- Any pending studies or overnight lab tests and trends of lab results. Also include certain criteria to act on (i.e., transfuse 1 unit PRBC if Hct is <28.
- Code status: This must be specified.
- Highlight any worrisome patients and why you are concerned. Include suggestions on how to deal with certain problems and what worked earlier in the hospital course.

Other Notes of Importance

10

. . . The paper chase . . .

OFF-SERVICE NOTES

. . . Passing the buck . . .

It is your final day on the floors, you've had a grueling month, and the last thing you want to do is write yet another note, let alone think about writing long, drawn-out off-service notes. However, the availability of concise off-service notes can be a life-saver to the intern coming onto the service. The following information is essential:

1. Date of admission.
2. Any new diagnoses/alterations in previous diagnoses.
3. Pertinent past medical history.
4. Hospital course (major interventions, events, procedures); this can be organized chronologically or by organ system depending on the patient. This is not a day-by-day recap of every test performed. Distill the story down to its essential details.
5. Current medications including day number for antibiotics.
6. Current pertinent PE and lab results.
7. Assessment and plan, including goals of care, and discharge needs (skilled nursing facility placement, home IV antibiotics, etc.).

PROCEDURE NOTES

. . . See one, do one, document one . . .

Procedural notes are of vital importance as part of the documentation of the hospital course and should include the following items:

1. Procedure, site of procedure. Regulatory bodies now require documentation of a pre-procedure "time-out" to announce the patient's name, and procedure performed.

2. Indication(s).
3. Consent.
4. Sterile prep used.
5. Anesthesia used.
6. Brief description of the procedure.
7. Specimens and what they were sent for.
8. Complications.
9. Postprocedure disposition and pending follow-up studies (i.e., CXR post-central line placement).

Any fluids that you just spent your valuable time collecting should be hand delivered to the lab personally (e.g., CSF, ABG, other taps, etc.).

DEATH/EXPIRATIONS

. . . The celestial discharge . . .

Interns are called on quite frequently to pronounce a death. Certain steps must be performed.

- On arrival to the bedside, you should observe for respirations, auscultate for heart sounds, palpate for a pulse, and attempt to elicit a corneal reflex. You also need to agree on an exact time of death with the nursing staff.
- Notify the private physician and family immediately, even in the middle of the night. The family must be asked specifically about (1) autopsy, (2) anatomic gift donation, and (3) funeral home. Appropriate forms for an autopsy and anatomic gifts must be completed. **Note:** Many hospitals have specially trained personnel to handle these particular requests, so be aware that it may not be appropriate for you to approach the family regarding these issues. Notify the appropriate hospital personnel if necessary.
- Complete a death note in the progress note section of the chart. It should include the following information: "Called by nursing to see patient regarding unresponsiveness. The patient was found to be breathless, pulseless, and without heart tones, blood pressure, and corneal reflexes. The patient was pronounced dead at 5:25 AM on August 29th, 2007. The patient's private physician and family were notified. The patient's family refused both anatomic gifts and

autopsy. The funeral home will be Manchester Mortuary." The word *dead* must be used.

- The Certificate of Death must be completed, including your assessment of cause of death. If the patient has a private physician, the death certificate will be completed by the private physician. Also, dictate a short death summary at this time.

Discharges

11

. . . Happy Trails! Come back if you have to . . .

With proper planning, discharges can be smooth for you and the patient. In today's environment, many more diseases are being managed and followed in the outpatient setting. Therefore, it is critical that the patient has follow-up and the patient's physician is aware of any pending issues and studies, or laboratory draws and imaging scheduled prior to outpatient follow-up. Communication with all involved parties is crucial to a successful discharge process. It also prevents many "bounce backs."

DISCHARGE PROCESS/PEARLS

- Obtain social work/case coordinator assistance early in the admission. Try to anticipate issues and problems early on (e.g., transportation, home oxygen, home antibiotics, or nursing/rehabilitation facility placement).
- Make sure the patient and his or her family is aware of possible discharge dates so they can arrange their schedules and not be caught off guard.
- Arrange for home services at least 24 hours before discharge (i.e., home nursing, home laboratory draws, PT, OT, etc.).
  - Criteria for home O_2:

    $PaO_2 < 55$ mm Hg

    PaO_2 of 55–59 mm Hg with evidence of cor pulmonale or secondary polycythemia (Hct >55%)

    O_2 sat < 88% on room air consistently (at rest, with exercise, or with sleep)

- Get rid of Foley catheters, sitters, telemetry monitoring, and supplemental oxygen as soon as possible. Many rehabilitation facilities require that these are not present 24 hours before discharge.
- Change antibiotics to PO the day before discharge. Avoid AM lab work the morning of discharge, unless absolutely necessary.

- Provide 1-month supply of all prescription medications, excluding controlled substances unless absolutely necessary. Reconcile discharge medications with admission medications. This paperwork can often be done in advance.
- Dictate the discharge summary at the time of discharge. It may seem painful at the time, but it will save you time later and prevent frustration on outpatient follow-up. It is most efficient to dictate when you are most familiar with the patient and hospital course. Take the extra 5–10 minutes to complete it now.
- The hospital course section of a well-organized discharge summary is generally organized by problem list.

DISCHARGE SUMMARY

Each institution has its own rules on discharge summaries. However, most should include the following items:

- Your name, the attending physician's name, and patient name and number.
- Date of admission and discharge.
- Principal and secondary diagnoses and procedures.
- Chief complaint, HPI, and allergies.
- Hospital course, including all major events, listing of major radiological and diagnostic test and results, and all major therapeutic interventions.
- Discharge medications, diet, and activity.
- Follow-up plans, including dates and times of outpatient appointments/studies.
- Condition on discharge.
- Copy distribution.

Top Ten Workups

12

CHEST PAIN

> . . . You may start to develop chest pain of your own . . .

Of course, angina or MI is your first thought. However, the most
important tool in identifying the cause of chest pain is a good history.
The patient should be assessed immediately.

Before you hang up the phone, ask the nurse for vital signs. Initial
verbal orders should include STAT ECG; O_2 by NC to keep saturations >92%; sublingual nitroglycerin 0.4 mg and aspirin 325 mg to
bedside. Confirm IV access.

Major Causes of Chest Pain

- Heart/vascular: Angina, MI, acute pericarditis, aortic dissection.
- Lungs: Pneumonia, PE, pneumothorax.
- GI: Esophageal spasm, GERD, PUD, pancreatitis.
- Other: Costochondritis, herpes zoster.

Things You Don't Want to Miss (Call Your Resident)

MI

Aortic dissection

PE

Pneumothorax

Key History

- Check BP, pulse, respirations, O_2 saturations, and chest pain.
- Quickly review chart.
- Take a focused history including quality, duration, radiation, changes
  with respiration, diaphoresis, and N/V.
- Review ECG. If cardiac etiology is suspected, give NTG SL if SBP
  >90. Also, make patient chew the aspirin, if not already given during
  the day.

Focused Examination

	KEY POINTS
General	How distressed or sick does the patient look?
Vitals	Hypotension is an ominous sign. Tachycardia may be from a PE or from pain. Bradycardia may be from AV block with inferior MI. Take BP in both arms to evaluate for aortic dissection. Fever may raise suspicion for PE.
Chest	Check for chest wall tenderness and any skin lesions. Listen for murmur, rubs, or gallops. Assess JVP.
Lungs	Assess for crackles, absent breath sounds on one side, friction rub.
Abdomen	Tenderness, bowel sounds.
Extremities	Edema or evidence of deep venous thrombosis. Examine pulses bilaterally in both upper and lower extremities to assess for aortic dissection.

Laboratory Data

Obtain an ECG if you haven't already done so. Review telemetry, if available. Check ABG if respiratory distress or low saturations are present; serial troponins (q12h × 2), portable CXR. Consider V/Q scan or spiral CT scan if PE is suspected; also consider lower extremity Dopplers. Consider contrast CT or TEE if aortic dissection is suspected.

Management

- **Cardiac:** If evidence of acute MI on ECG (ST elevation of 1 mm or more in two contiguous leads or new LBBB) and history, call a STAT cardiology consult for consideration of reperfusion therapy (thrombolytics or angioplasty). Ensure the patient is on a monitor, has IV access, has oxygen 2 L by NC, and has received an aspirin. Consider administering β-blockers, nitrates, morphine, heparin (LMWH or UFH). Consider loading with clopidogrel, 300 mg PO, and starting a glycoprotein IIb/IIIa inhibitor (e.g., eptifibatide or tirofiban). Metoprolol, 5 mg IV, may be initiated and repeated every 5 minutes for a total dose of 15 mg.
- **Angina:** NTG SL, 0.4 mg times 3 every 5 minutes, assuming SBP >90. Consider β-blockers, IV or transdermal NTG, heparin, and antiplatelet agents. Place on telemetry. If patient is still having chest pain after NTG SL times 3, consider giving morphine and starting NTG drip to titrate until chest pain free.
- **Aortic dissection:** Arrange for immediate transfer to CCU/MICU. Start nitroprusside or labetalol for BP control. STAT vascular/thoracic surgery consult.

- *Pulmonary:* If PE, ensure adequate oxygenation and administer LMWH or UFH. See Therapeutics section for dosing (Chapter 15).

- *Pneumothorax:* Tension pneumothorax requires immediate needle decompression in the second intercostal space in the midclavicular line, followed by chest tube. Other pneumothoraces involving >20% of the lung require a surgery consult for chest tube placement.

- *GI:* Antacids such as aluminum hydroxide (Maalox), 30 mL PO prn q4–6h (avoid in patients with renal failure), famotidine (Pepcid), 20 mg PO bid, or omeprazole (Prilosec), 20 mg PO q day. Elevate the head of the bed, especially after meals.

Refractory Chest Pain

- Reevaluate patient for causes of chest pain—has your initial impression changed?
- Repeat ECG, vital signs, physical exam.
- For ongoing cardiac ischemia, particularly with elevated troponins and/or ST segment depression, start a NTG drip, consider further antiplatelet agent therapy, and consider an urgent cardiology consult.

ABDOMINAL PAIN

. . . Not just from the cafeteria food . . .

What are the patient's vital signs? How severe is the pain? Is this a new problem? If vital signs are stable, inform the nurse you will be there shortly and to call you immediately if things worsen before you arrive.

Major Causes of Abdominal Pain

Figure 12-1 list some causes of abdominal pain by location. Generalized abdominal pain may be due to various causes such as: appendicitis (at its inception); intestinal infection, inflammation, ischemia, and obstruction; peritonitis of any cause; diabetic ketoacidosis; sickle cell crisis; acute intermittent porphyria; ruptured aneurysm, and acute adrenocortical insufficiency.

Things You Don't Want to Miss (Call Your Resident)

AAA rupture

Bowel rupture, perforation, or ischemia

Ascending cholangitis

Acute appendicitis

Retroperitoneal hematoma

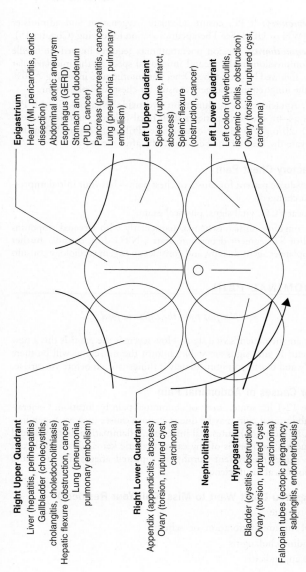

Epigastrium
Heart (MI, pericarditis, aortic dissection)
Abdominal aortic aneurysm
Esophagus (GERD)
Stomach and duodenum (PUD, cancer)
Pancreas (pancreatitis, cancer)
Lung (pneumonia, pulmonary embolism)

Left Upper Quadrant
Spleen (rupture, infarct, abscess)
Splenic flexure (obstruction, cancer)

Left Lower Quadrant
Left colon (diverticulitis, ischemic colitis, obstruction)
Ovary (torsion, ruptured cyst, carcinoma)

Right Upper Quadrant
Liver (hepatitis, perihepatitis)
Gallbladder (cholecystitis, cholangitis, choledocholithiasis)
Hepatic flexure (obstruction, cancer)
Lung (pneumonia, pulmonary embolism)

Right Lower Quadrant
Appendix (appendicitis, abscess)
Ovary (torsion, ruptured cyst, carcinoma)

Nephrolithiasis

Hypogastrium
Bladder (cystitis, obstruction)
Ovary (torsion, ruptured cyst, carcinoma)
Fallopian tubes (ectopic pregnancy, salpingitis, endometriosis)

Figure 12-1 Major causes of abdominal pain.

Key History

- Check BP, pulse, respirations, O_2 saturations, and temperature.
- Quickly look at the patient and review the chart.
- Take a focused history, including quality, duration, radiation, changes with respiration, location, N/V (bilious versus nonbilious), last bowel movement, and any hematemesis, melena, or hematochezia. For women of childbearing age, ask about their last menstrual period.
- Mesenteric ischemia often has pain out of proportion to examination. Consider this, especially with a history of atrial fibrillation, vascular disease, and in elderly patients.

Focused Examination

KEY POINTS

General	How distressed or sick does the patient look?
Vitals	Repeat now, especially BP.
HEENT	Check for icterus.
Chest	Check for any skin lesions. Listen for murmur, rubs, or gallops. Assess JVP.
Lungs	Assess for crackles, absent breath sounds on one side, friction rub.
Abdomen	Inspect bowel sounds: high pitched with SBO, absent with ileus. Percussion: tympany, shifting dullness. Palpation: guarding, rebound tenderness, Murphy's sign, psoas, and obturator signs. Assess for CVA tenderness.
Rectal	Must be performed. Guaiac for occult blood.
Pelvic	If indicated by history.

Laboratory Data

Consider CBC, electrolytes, ABG, lactate, LFTs, amylase, lipase, β-hCG, and UA. Films to consider include flat and upright abdominal films, CXR, and ECG. Abdominal CT, ultrasound, or both may be required.

Management

- The initial goal is to determine if the patient has an acute abdomen and needs surgical evaluation and treatment. Avoid any analgesics as this may mask the pain and obscure the evaluation. An acute abdomen includes such signs as rebound tenderness or guarding and conditions such as ruptured viscus, abscess, or hemorrhage. (See Acute Abdomen under the General Surgery consult section in Chapter 17.)

- Other conditions can be managed using a more detailed and leisurely approach, after the acute abdomen has been ruled out.
- Keep the patient NPO. Ensure large bore IV access and run maintenance fluids.

ACUTE ALTERED MENTAL STATUS

. . . Not unlike your post-call . . .

What are the patient's vital signs? What was the time course of changes? Any change in level of consciousness or any trauma? Is the patient a diabetic? Does the patient have a cardiac history? Any recent narcotics or sedatives given? What was the reason for admission (e.g., alcohol or drug intoxication/withdrawal)?

Initial verbal orders to consider: think of TONG (thiamine, oxygen, naloxone, and glucose). Have the nurse obtain Accucheck and oxygen saturations now.

Acute mental status changes associated with fever or decreased consciousness require that you see the patient immediately.

Major Causes of Acute Altered Mental Status
Think *DELIRIUMS*:

D = Drug effect or withdrawal (e.g., EtOH; narcs, benzos, anticholinergics, etc.; especially in the elderly, even in low doses)

E = Emotional (e.g., anxiety, pain)

L = Low PO_2 (e.g., MI, PE, anemia) or high PCO_2 (e.g., COPD)

I = Infection

R = Retention of urine or feces

I = Ictal states

U = Undernutrition/Underhydration

M = Metabolic (lytes, glucose, thyroid, liver, kidney)

S = Subdural (acute CNS processes, e.g., head trauma, hematoma, hydrocephalus, CVA/TIA)

Things You Don't Want to Miss (Call Your Resident)
Sepsis or meningitis
Intracranial mass or increased pressure
Alcohol withdrawal (DTs)
Acute CVA

Key History
- Check BP, pulse, respirations, O_2 saturations, temperature, and Accucheck.
- Quickly look at the patient and review the chart.
- Confirm no falls or trauma.
- Review chart for new meds or narcotics.
- Take a focused history, including onset and level of responsiveness.

Focused Examination

	KEY POINTS
General	How distressed or sick does the patient look?
HEENT	Look for signs of trauma; pupil size, symmetry, and response to light; papilledema and nuchal rigidity.
Chest	Check for any skin lesions. Listen for murmur, rubs, or gallops.
Lungs	Assess for crackles, equal breath sounds.
Abdomen	Look for ascites, jaundice, and other signs of liver disease.
Neurologic	Thoroughly examine, including mental status examination, and check for asterixis.

Laboratory Data
Consider CBC, electrolytes, LFTs, ABG, TSH, ammonia level, UA, cultures, ECG, and CXR. Other studies that may be required are lumbar puncture, CT, and EEG. The performance of a head CT before lumbar puncture is controversial but is generally not required for nonelderly, immunocompetent patients who present without focal neurologic abnormalities, seizures, or diminished level of consciousness.

Management
- Management is based on findings on examination and laboratory data. If meningitis is suspected, lumbar puncture should be performed as detailed above. In addition, empiric antibiotics should be started STAT (see Chapter 17, Neurology consult section for antibiotic choices).
- Alcohol withdrawal needs to be treated urgently with benzodiazepines, usually with chlordiazepoxide (Librium) 50–100 mg PO q6–8h or lorazepam (Ativan) 0.5–1 mg PO/IV/IM q6–8h (prn or scheduled). Thiamine, 100 mg IV/IM, should also be administered, especially before any glucose. See Chapter 13 for further management strategies.

ACUTE RENAL FAILURE

. . . Like you have time to use the bathroom . . .

What are the patient's vital signs? How much urine has been produced in the last 24 hours? In the last 8 hours? Does the patient have a Foley catheter inserted? What are the patient's recent electrolytes, especially potassium, BUN, creatinine, and bicarbonate?

If the patient does have a Foley catheter inserted, ask the nurse to flush the catheter with 30 mL NS. If the patient does not have a Foley catheter, ask the nurse to place one now. Tell the nurse you will see the patient shortly.

Major Causes of Oliguria

Oliguria is generally defined as <500 mL of urine per 24 hours. Major causes of oliguria can be broken down as follows:

- **Prerenal:** Volume depletion, congestive heart failure, vascular occlusion.
- **Renal:** Glomerular, tubular/interstitial (acute tubular necrosis caused by drugs or toxins), and vascular.
- **Postrenal:** Obstruction (BPH), clogged Foley catheter, stones.

Things You Don't Want to Miss (Call Your Resident)

Hyperkalemia

Severe acidosis

Acute, marked uremia

Life-threatening volume overload

Key History

- Check BP, pulse, respirations, O_2 saturations, and temperature.
- Quickly look at the patient and review the chart.
- Take a focused history.
- Determining volume status is important. Review ins and outs over the past few days. Any new medications (e.g., ACE inhibitors, diuretics, NSAIDs, IV contrast dye)?

Focused Examination

	KEY POINTS
General	How distressed or sick does the patient look?
Vitals	Check orthostatics and weight over the past few days.

Cardiovascular	Check for JVD, friction rub, and skin turgor.
Abdomen	Look for ascites or enlarged bladder.
Genitourinary	Check for enlarged prostate.
Extremities	Assess perfusion. Check for asterixis.

Laboratory Data

UA: Look for cells, casts, protein. Consider serum electrolytes, urine electrolytes, calculate FENa (and/or FEurea), urine eosinophils, ABG, and ECG. Renal ultrasound should be ordered within 24 hours to rule out hydronephrosis and evaluate the renal system.

Management

- The minimum acceptable urine output is 30 mL/hr. If flushing the Foley catheter did not help, ask the nurse to change the Foley catheter.
- Initial management should be directed at treating life-threatening electrolyte disorders and correcting volume contraction and hypotension. Obtain diagnostic urinary studies before administering diuretics. Don't forget to adjust drug doses based on glomerular filtration rate.
- Calculate the fractional excretion of sodium:

$$FENa = U[Na] \times P[Cr]/U[Cr] \times P[Na]$$

This equation is most useful with oliguric renal failure but may be helpful in nonoliguric renal failure. FENa >1% to 2% with oliguria is almost always ATN but can be prerenal with diuretics. FENa <1% with oliguria is generally prerenal: volume depletion, severe CHF, or nephrotic syndrome, NSAID or dye toxicity, sepsis, cyclosporine toxicity, acute GN, and hepatorenal syndrome. Calculate FEurea in nonoliguric renal failure or if diuretics have been given. FEurea <35% is consistent with prerenal state.

- If hyperkalemia is suspected, order an ECG and STAT serum potassium.
- A STAT renal consult is required if the patient needs urgent dialysis. Indications for urgent dialysis include *AEIOU*, where: A = Acidemia (pH <7.2)

> E = Electrolyte disorder (e.g., hyperkalemia when unable to manage medically–see Chapter 13).
>
> I = Intoxication (e.g., alcohol, salicylates, theophylline, lithium, etc.).

O = Overload (e.g., pulmonary edema when unable to manage medically).

U = Uremia (encephalopathy, pericarditis).

- **Prerenal causes** can be initially managed with a small volume challenge, such as 250–500 mL NS bolus depending on the cardiovascular status of the patient. This can be followed by NS at a set rate. Specific criteria should be given to the nursing staff (i.e., call HO if urine output is <30 mL/hr). Alternatively, if congestive heart failure is suspected, the patient may need diuresis. Escalating doses of furosemide (Lasix) can be used, and urine output and daily weights can be assessed. With a fluid challenge, the creatinine level often trends down by the next morning if the cause is prerenal.

- **Postrenal causes** can be potentially managed by placing a Foley catheter. If immediate flow is obtained, urethral obstruction is likely. If a Foley cannot be placed due to obstruction, consider a urology consultation.

- For **contrast-induced ARF prophylaxis**, euvolemia is essential. Use ½ NS or NS at 1 mg/kg/hr for 6–12 hours before and 6–12 hours after the procedure.

HEADACHE

. . . Like your head isn't pounding by now . . .

What are the patient's vital signs? How severe is the headache? Has there been a change in consciousness? Has the patient had similar headaches in the past? If so, what relieves them?

If the headache is severe and acute or associated with N/V, changes in vision, fever, or decreased consciousness, the patient should be seen immediately. Otherwise, inform the nurse you will see the patient shortly.

Major Causes of Headache
- Tension
- Vascular (migraine, subarachnoid hemorrhage)
- Cluster
- Drugs
- Temporal arteritis
- Infectious (meningitis, sinusitis)

- Trauma
- CVA
- Hypertension
- Mass lesions

Things You Don't Want to Miss (Call Your Resident)
Meningitis
Subarachnoid hemorrhage or subdural hematoma
Mass lesion associated with herniation

Key History
- Check BP, pulse, respirations, O_2 saturations, and temperature.
- Quickly look at the patient and review the chart.
- A detailed, well-focused history is the best method for evaluating a headache. Most are tension or migraine type, but more serious conditions need to be ruled out.

Focused Examination

KEY POINTS
General	How distressed or sick does the patient look?
HEENT	Look for signs of trauma, pupil size, symmetry, response to light, papilledema, nuchal rigidity, temporal artery tenderness, and sinus tenderness.
Neurologic	Thorough examination, including mental status.

Laboratory Data
Consider CBC and ESR if temporal arteritis suspected. Head CT should be considered for:

- A chronic headache pattern that has changed or a new severe headache occurs.
- A new headache in a patient older than 50 years.
- Focal findings on neurologic examination.

If meningitis is suspected, lumbar puncture should be performed. The performance of a head CT before lumbar puncture is controversial but is generally not required for nonelderly, immunocompetent patients who present without focal neurologic abnormalities, seizures or diminished level of consciousness.

Management

- The initial goal is to exclude the serious life-threatening conditions mentioned previously. After such conditions have been excluded, management can focus on symptomatic relief.
- For suspected bacterial meningitis, start antibiotics immediately. See Chapter 17, Neurology consult section for antibiotic choices.
- For suspected subdural hematoma or subarachnoid hemorrhage, obtain CT scan. If positive, a neurosurgery consultation should be obtained.
- Tension headaches and mild migraines can be treated with acetaminophen (Tylenol), 650–1,000 mg PO q6h prn or ibuprofen (Motrin), 200–600 mg PO q6–8h. Consider sumatriptan (Imitrex), 25 mg PO for moderate to severe migraine headaches; can repeat 25–100 mg q2h for maximum of 200–300 mg/day.
- Severe migraines may require a narcotic such as meperidine or codeine. Sumatriptan, or ergotamine, is usually most effective in the prodromal stage. These agents are contraindicated in patients with angina, uncontrolled hypertension, hemiplegia, or basilar artery migraine.

HYPOTENSION AND HYPERTENSION

. . . Too high, too low, uh oh . . .

Hypotension

What are the patient's vital signs? Is the patient conscious, confused, or disoriented? What has the patient's blood pressure been? What was the reason for admission?

If impending or established shock is suspected, ensure IV access (at least 20 gauge IV) and have the patient placed in Trendelenburg's position (head of bed down). Hypotension requires that you see the patient immediately.

Major Causes of Hypotension
- Cardiogenic (rate or pump problem)
- Hypovolemic
- Septic shock
- Anaphylaxis

Things You Don't Want to Miss (Call Your Resident)
Shock, which is evidence of inadequate perfusion. This is best assessed by looking at end organs: brain (mental status), heart (chest pain), kidneys

(urine output), and skin (cool, clammy). Shock is a clinical diagnosis defined as a systolic BP <90, with evidence of inadequate tissue perfusion.

Key History
- Check BP (both arms), pulse, respirations, O_2 saturations, and temperature.
- Quickly look at the patient and review chart. Get an ECG.

Focused Examination

KEY POINTS

General	How distressed or sick does the patient look?
Vitals	Repeat now. Elevated temperature and hypotension suggest sepsis.
Neurologic	Mentation.
Cardiovascular	Heart rate, JVP, skin temperature, color, and warmth. Capillary refill.
Lungs	Listen for crackles, breath sounds on both sides.
GI	Any evidence of blood loss?

Laboratory Data
Consider troponins, ECG, ABG, CBC, electrolytes, and CXR.

Management
- Examine the ECG and take the pulse yourself. Check BP in both arms. A compensatory sinus tachycardia is an expected appropriate response to hypotension. However, check the ECG to ensure that the patient does not have atrial fibrillation, SVT, or ventricular tachycardia, which may cause hypotension because of decreased diastolic filling. Bradycardia may be seen in autonomic dysfunction or heart block.
- Most causes of shock require fluids to normalize the intravascular volume. Use normal saline or lactated Ringer's. The exception is cardiogenic shock, which may require preload and afterload reduction, inotropic and/or vasopressor support, and transfer to an ICU.
- Hypovolemic, anaphylactic, and septic shock require fluids. Use boluses of 500 mL to 1 L. If no response, repeat bolus or leave fluids open.
- Anaphylactic shock requires epinephrine, 0.3 mg IV immediately and repeated every 10–15 minutes as required. Hydrocortisone, 500 mg IV, and diphenhydramine (Benadryl), 25 mg IV, should also be administered.

- In septic shock, IV fluids and antibiotics can resolve the shock. However, continuing hypotension requires ICU admission for vasopressors.
- Cardiogenic shock can be the result of an acute MI or worsening CHF. However, other causes of hypotension and elevated JVP include acute cardiac tamponade, PE, and tension pneumothorax. These always need to be considered.

Hypertension

. . . Feel YOUR blood pressure rising? . . .

What are the patient's vital signs? What has the patient's blood pressure been? What is the reason for admission? What BP medications has the patient been taking? Does the patient have signs of hypertensive emergency?

The rate of rise of the BP and the setting in which the high BP is occurring are more important than the level of BP itself. Elevated blood pressure alone, in the absence of symptoms or new or progressive target organ damage, rarely requires emergent therapy.

Hypertensive emergencies require that you see the patient immediately. Make sure the patient has an IV and order an ECG. Inform the nurse that you will arrive shortly.

Hypertensive Emergencies
- Encephalopathy
- Intracranial hemorrhage
- Unstable angina or MI
- Acute left ventricular failure with pulmonary edema
- Aortic dissection
- Eclampsia
- Renal insufficiency (new or worsened)

Hypertensive Urgencies
- Blood pressure >180/110
- Optic disc edema
- Severe perioperative hypertension

Things You Don't Want to Miss (Call Your Resident)
Hypertensive emergencies

Key History
- Check BP, pulse, respirations, O_2 saturations, and temperature.
- Quickly look at the patient and review the chart. Get an ECG.

Focused Examination

KEY POINTS

General	How distressed or sick does the patient look?
Vitals	Repeat BP now in both arms.
Neurologic	Mentation, confusion, delirium, focal neurologic deficits.
HEENT	Fundi for papilledema, retinal hemorrhages, or hypertensive changes.
Cardiovascular	Heart rate, jugular venous pulse, color. Capillary refill.
Lungs	Listen for crackles, breath sounds on both sides.

Laboratory Data

Consider troponins, ECG, ABG, CBC, electrolytes, UA, and CXR.

Management

- Treat the patient, not the BP reading. Acute lowering of BP of asymptomatic patients with long-standing hypertension can be dangerous.

- Hypertensive emergencies require an ICU setting. The goal is to reduce the MAP by no more than 25% in the first 2 hours. IV hydralazine, nitroprusside, labetalol, or enalaprilat are often used. While arranging transfer to the ICU, certain wards allow medications to be started. Consider IV nitroglycerin for hypertension associated with MI or pulmonary edema. Nitroprusside and labetolol are useful in aortic dissection. Nitroprusside is also used for patients with encephalopathy but often requires intra-arterial blood pressure monitoring.

- Hypertensive urgencies can usually be managed with oral medications with the goal of reducing BP over 24–48 hours. Examples include captopril, 25–50 mg PO, clonidine, 0.1–0.2 mg PO, or labetalol, 200–400 mg PO. These can be repeated or titrated every 2–4 hours. Close follow-up is essential.

COMMON ARRHYTHMIAS

. . . Too fast, too slow, or too irregular . . .

What are the patient's vital signs, including temperature? Any chest pain or shortness of breath?

Order a STAT ECG. Patients with chest pain, shortness of breath, or hypotension need to be seen immediately.

Major Causes of Rapid Heart Rate and Slow Rates
- Rapid rates

  Regular: sinus tachycardia, SVT, ventricular tachycardia, atrial flutter

  Irregular: atrial fibrillation, multifocal atrial tachycardia
- Slow rates

  Drugs (β-blockers, CCB, digoxin)

  Sick sinus syndrome

  MI (especially inferior)

  AV block

Things You Don't Want to Miss (Call Your Resident)
Ventricular tachycardia

Hypotension

Angina or MI

Key History
- Check BP, pulse, respirations, O_2 saturations, and temperature.
- Quick look at patient and quick review of chart. Get an ECG.

Focused Examination

	KEY POINTS
General	How distressed or sick does the patient look?
Vitals	Repeat now.
Neurologic	Mentation.
Cardiovascular	Heart rate, jugular venous pulse, skin temperature and color, capillary refill.
Lungs	Listen for crackles and breath sounds on both sides.

Laboratory Data
Consider troponins, ECG, ABG, CBC, electrolytes, and CXR.

Management
- Always complete the ABCs first and ensure O_2, and IV access. Place patient on monitor or telemetry; consider transfer to a monitored bed on a cardiology floor.
- If patient is hypotensive and has atrial fibrillation with RVR, SVT, or ventricular tachycardia, emergency cardioversion may be required.

- In general, if the patient is unstable with serious signs or symptoms, a ventricular rate greater than 150, or both, you should prepare for immediate cardioversion. The patient may require sedation—call your resident. Serious signs and symptoms per ACLS protocol include chest pain, shortness of breath, decreased level of consciousness, hypotension and shock, congestive heart failure, and acute MI. Refer to the proper ACLS algorithm at this point (see Chapter 2) and call your resident.

- Atrial fibrillation with rapid rate but without evidence of hemodynamic compromise can be rate controlled with diltiazem, metoprolol, or digoxin. Amiodarone can also be considered, though there is a risk of pharmacologic cardioversion. See ECG section (Chapter 16) for dosing.

- SVT without evidence of hemodynamic compromise can some-times be broken with Valsalva maneuver, carotid sinus massage (one side at a time and always listen for bruits first), or both. If still in SVT, try adenosine, 6 mg rapid IV push, followed by 12 mg rapid IV push if necessary. Always remember to flush with at least 20 mL of 0.9 NS after each IV push. If the complex width is narrow with stable BP, verapamil, 2.5–5 mg IV, or diltiazem, 10 mg IV, can be used. If wide complex, manage as stable VT.

- For ventricular tachycardia, if pulseless or without BP, manage as ventricular fibrillation. If ventricular tachycardia with serious signs or symptoms, consider immediate synchronized cardioversion. If stable, follow the ACLS protocol (see Chapter 2).

FEVER

. . . Of known or unknown origin . . .

What are the patient's vital signs? What was the reason for admission? Is this a new finding? Any associated symptoms (e.g., cough, headache, change in mental status, N/V, and so forth)? Any antipyretics or cur-rent antibiotics? Any recent surgeries (think of postoperative fever)?

Order blood and urine cultures. Patients with meningitis symp-toms or hypotension need to be seen immediately.

Major Causes of Fever

- Infections: Best to think of by site—lung, urine, IV sites, blood, CNS, abdomen and pelvis, GI; consider immune status
- Drug-induced fever: Many drugs have been implicated
- Atelectasis (especially post-op)
- Neoplasms
- Connective tissue diseases

- Deep venous thrombosis/pulmonary embolism
- Fever of unknown origin

Things You Don't Want To Miss
Meningitis
Septic shock

Key History
- Check BP, pulse, respirations, O_2 saturations, and temperature.
- Quickly look at the patient and review the chart.

Focused Examination

	KEY POINTS
General	How distressed or sick does the patient look? Check all catheter sites (IV, central line, Foley, G-tube, etc.).
Vitals	Repeat now. Tachycardia is an expected finding with fever. Recheck blood pressure.
Neurologic	Mentation, photophobia, neck stiffness, Brudzinski's or Kernig's signs.
Cardiovascular	Heart rate, jugular venous pulse, skin temperature and color. Any new murmurs? Capillary refill.
Lungs	Listen for crackles and breath sounds on both sides.
Abdomen	Assess for RUQ tenderness and bowel sounds.
Extremities	Check calves for signs of deep venous thrombosis, joints for effusions.

Laboratory Data
Consider CBC, blood cultures (two sets at different sites; if a central line is present, be sure to get one peripheral set as well), CMP, UA and culture, sputum culture and Gram's stain, CXR. LP if meningitis is suspected. Consider *Clostridium difficile* stool cultures.

Management
- Make sure the patient is hemodynamically stable. Review medications and obtain cultures. Give antipyretics (acetaminophen 650 mg PO/PR or ibuprofen 400 mg PO q6–8 hours PRN). Ensure IV access and consider maintenance fluids, including insensible losses.

- Consider antibiotics. If the patient is hemodynamically stable, immunocompetent, not toxic appearing, with no clear source of infection, it may be prudent to withhold antibiotics and recheck cultures.
- Patients with fever and hypotension require broad-spectrum antibiotics and IV fluids or pressors to manage the hypotension. Septic shock is an emergency. (Please refer to Hypotension Management earlier in this chapter.)
- Patients with fever and neutropenia (<500 cells/mm^3) require a careful physical examination, with particular attention paid to mucosal surfaces, lungs, skin, and vascular access sites. Blood cultures for bacteria and fungi should be drawn; also consider urine culture, sputum culture, LP, and CXR if clinically indicated. Broad spectrum antibiotics should be started. Choices for initial therapy include cefepime, ceftazidime, carbapenem, or an antipseudomonal penicillin, with or without aminoglycoside. If a catheter-related infection is suspected or the patient is known to be colonized with penicillin-resistant pneumococcus or methicillin-resistant *S. aureus*, consider adding vancomycin to the above regimen.
- Patients with fever and meningitis symptoms require antibiotics immediately. Do not wait for the LP kit. Give the antibiotics, then approach the LP.
- Consider changing or removing Foley catheters and any indwelling IV sites.

Febrile Neutropenia

NOTE: The following recommendations are based on antibiotic resistance patterns specific to Barnes Jewish Hospital (adapted from Barnes Jewish Hospital Stem Cell Transplant Unit Febrile Neutropenia Pathway, Barnes-Jewish Hospital Department of Pharmacy, Washington University Medical Center, 2007). Consult your hospital's antibiogram to tailor antimicrobial therapy to local resistance patterns.

Definition
Fever >38.3°C, or ≥38.1°C for at least 1 hour, with ANC ≤ 500 or anticipate ANC to fall <500:

A. Work-up: Obtain blood cultures ×2, physical exam, chest x-ray, UA, and culture.

B. Initial Treatment:

    1. Cefepime 1 g IV q8h. *If PCN Allergy: ciprofloxacin 400 mg IV q12h or aztreonam 2 g IV q8h.*

2. Vancomycin 1 g IV q12h if any of the following are present:
   a. Severe mucositis.
   b. Clinical evidence of catheter-related infection.
   c. Known colonization with resistant streptococcus or staphylococcus.
   d. Sudden temperature spike >40°C.
   e. Hypotension or sepsis.
3. Consider metronidazole 500 mg IV q8h, if suspected oropharyngeal or intra-abdominal source.
4. Consider addition of gentamycin 5 mg/kg IV q24h, if clinically unstable.
5. Tailor antibiotics based on culture results.

C. Treatment of persistent fevers: *new fever after afebrile ≥48 hours or persistently febrile ≥72 hours and cultures negative.*
   1. If clinically unstable: change GNR coverage to meropenem 500 mg IV q6h or ciprofloxacin 400 mg IV q12h ± aminoglycoside.
   2. If clinically stable: continue current regimen and tailor based on cultures results.
   3. If persistently febrile >5 days and cultures negative:
      a. If patient *not* on antimold prophylaxis and *no* identified clinical sites suspicious for fungal infection: use echindocandin.
      b. If patient *not* on antimold prophylaxis and clinical site suspicious for fungal infection ***excluding sinusitis*** (see below): use voriconazole, weight-based dosing for IV and PO administration.
      c. If patient on antimold prophylaxis and *no* identified clinical sites suspicious for fungal infection:
         i. Clinically stable: no change in antifungals, monitor closely.
         ii. Clinically unstable: amphotericin B lipid complex (ABLC) 5 mg/kg IV q day. *If already receiving amphotericin product, obtain an ID consult for antifungal selection.*
      d. If patient on antimold prophylaxis and clinical site suspicious for fungal infection: use ABLC 5 mg/kg IV q day.
      e. It patient has suspected fungal sinusitis: ABLC 5 mg/kg IV q day.

D. Antibiotics:

  1. Discontinue vancomycin after 72 hours if cultures negative for coagulase negative staphylococci, oxacillin-resistant *S. aureus*, cephalosporin-resistant streptococci, or *C. jeikeium*.

  2. Discontinue double GNR coverage (e.g., aminogylcoside) after 72 hours if cultures negative for GNR and patient clinically stable.

  3. Culture negative for 3–5 days.

   a. Afebrile and ANC ≥500, discontinue after 48 hours.

   b. Afebrile and ANC <500, continue antibiotics until ANC ≥500 for 48 hours.

   c. Febrile and ANC ≥500, reassess after 4–5 days.

   d. Febrile and ANC <500, continue antibiotics until neutropenia resolves.

  4. Culture positive

   a. Remove line if *Pseudomonas, Stenotrophomonas, Acinetobacter*, VRE, *S. aureus, C. jeikeium*, and *Candida*.

   b. For all other organisms and tunnel catheter infections, consider removing line.

   c. Continue antibiotics until ANC ≥500 × 7 days or for 14 days, whichever is longer.

  5. UTI: continue until ANC is ≥500.

  6. Pneumonia

   a. Bacterial: until ANC ≥500 × 7 days or for 14 days, whichever is longer.

   b. *Aspergillus* (suspected or proven): Voriconazole (weight-based dosing) and consider ID consult.

SHORTNESS OF BREATH

. . . You were in good physical shape . . .

What are the patient's vital signs, including temperature? When was the onset of SOB and what was the reason for admission? Does the patient have COPD or is the patient getting oxygen?

Order oxygen and an ABG kit to the bedside. Patients with SOB need to be seen immediately.

Major Causes of Shortness of Breath
- Pulmonary: Asthma, COPD, pulmonary embolism, pneumonia
- Cardiovascular: CHF, cardiac tamponade
- Others: Pneumothorax, obstruction (e.g., mucous plug), anxiety

Things You Don't Want to Miss (Call Your Resident)
Inadequate tissue oxygenation (i.e., hypoxia)

Tension pneumothorax

Airway obstruction

Key History
- Check BP, pulse, respirations, O_2 saturations, and temperature.
- Quickly look at the patient and review the chart. Get an ECG, ABG, and CXR if the patient looks sick.

Focused Examination

	KEY POINTS
General	How distressed or sick does the patient look?
Vitals	Repeat now. Check for a pulsus paradoxus.
Neurologic	Mentation and check for central cyanosis.
Cardiovascular	Heart rate, jugular venous pulse, skin temperature and color, capillary refill.
Lungs	Listen for crackles and breath sounds on both sides, evidence of consolidation or effusion.

Laboratory Data
Consider ABG, ECG, troponins, CBC, D-dimer, V/Q scan, and CXR. If you have any doubt at all, get an ABG—if you think about it you should do it. Beware of relying on pulse oximetry alone.

Management
- Order empiric oxygen to keep saturations >92%. Be cautious if the patient has COPD and is a retainer of CO_2—in that case, keep O_2 saturations around 88% to 90% and check ABG. Remember that the O_2 saturation tells you nothing about pH or PCO_2.
- For asthma or COPD, administer albuterol and ipatropium by nebulizer, q2–4h until stable. Consider IV corticosteroids, methylprednisolone (Solu-Medrol), 60 mg IV q6h, and antibiotics if needed.

- For CHF, is the patient volume overloaded? Raise the head of the patient's bed. Administer furosemide (Lasix), 20–40 mg IV, and albuterol nebulizer. Consider morphine or nitroglycerin. Assess for adequate diuresis.
- For suspected cardiac tamponade, order a STAT cardiac echo and cardiology consult.
- For pulmonary embolism, often the patient is tachycardic and tachypneic and has a sudden onset of SOB. The classic, though not usually present, ECG findings are S_1, Q_3, and T_3 (S waves in lead I, Q waves in lead III, inverted T waves in lead III). If suspicion is high, consider starting heparin or LMWH. Ensure that the patient has no history of bleeding disorders, PUD, recent CVA, or surgery. Obtain a V/Q scan or spiral CT. Also, consider lower extremity Dopplers.
- Acute respiratory failure is generally defined by ABG of PO_2 <60 or PCO_2 >50 with a pH <7.3 while on room air. Ensure that the patient hasn't received narcotics recently. If so, consider naloxone, 0.2 mg IV. Acute respiratory acidosis with a pH <7.2 usually requires mechanical ventilation.

GASTROINTESTINAL BLEEDING

. . . Ahh, the smell of melena . . .

What are the patient's vital signs? When was the onset of bleeding and what is the reason for admission? Is the bleeding upper (coffee ground emesis, melena) or lower (hematochezia)? How much blood has been lost?

Confirm that the patient has IV access (at least 18 gauge) and recent CBC. Type and cross-match blood. If the patient is tachycardic or hypotensive, see the patient immediately.

Major Causes of Gastrointestinal Bleeding

- Upper: Esophageal varices, Mallory-Weiss tear, peptic ulcer, esophagitis, neoplasm, aortoenteric fistula (history of AAA repair)
- Lower: Diverticulosis, angiodysplasia, neoplasm, IBD, infectious colitis, anorectal disease (hemorrhoids, fissures)

Things You Don't Want to Miss (Call Your Resident)

GI bleeding leading to hypovolemic shock

Key History

• Check BP, pulse, respirations, O_2 saturations, and temperature. Orthostatic BP.
• Quickly look at the patient and review the chart.

Focused Examination

	KEY POINTS
General	How distressed or sick does the patient look?
Vitals	Repeat now.
Neurologic	Mentation.
HEENT	Check for conjunctival pallor.
Cardiovascular	Heart rate, jugular venous pulse, skin temperature and color, capillary refill.
Abdomen	Check for tenderness, bowel sounds, look for ascites.
Rectal	Must be performed. Guaiac stool.

Laboratory Data

Consider CBC, coags, and CMP.

Management

• Insert two large-bore IVs (16–18 gauge), type and cross pRBCs. It can take up to 8 hours for CBC to equilibrate, so initial Hct may be falsely elevated. In absence of renal disease, high BUN suggests GI bleeding. Check coags and platelets to exclude bleeding disorders. Is the patient receiving anticoagulants? If so, stop the anticoagulant and consider reversal with FFP or vitamin K.

• Consider whether special blood products are required based on comorbidities (e.g., irradiated, washed RBCs). Also consider whether the patient needs premedication with acetaminophen/diphenhydramine based on prior transfusions.

• Replenish the intravascular volume by giving IV fluids (normal saline), especially while awaiting blood products. Keep the patient NPO.

• For upper GI bleeding, insert a nasogastric tube to assess if active bleeding is present. Suppress acid with PO (or IV) proton pump inhibitor therapy. GI consult for endoscopy. If bleeding has stopped and the patient is hemodynamically stable, elective endoscopy can be performed within the next 24 hours. Otherwise, urgent endoscopy may be required.

- For active variceal bleeding, start IV octreotide, 50 μg bolus, then 50 μg/hour, correct coagulation deficits, replace pRBCs as needed. Call a GI consult as urgent endoscopy may be required.
- For lower GI bleeding, correct fluid status. If hemodynamically stable, obtain GI consult for colonoscopy. If unstable, an urgent tagged RBC scan should be scheduled. Also, consider arteriography.
- Surgery consult/indications include the following:
  - Aortoenteric fistula.
  - Uncontrollable or recurrent bleeding.
  - Bleeding episode requiring transfusion of more than 6 units pRBCs.
  - Visible naked vessel seen in peptic ulcer by endoscopy.

Common Calls and Complaints

13

. . . *You rang*. . .

ALCOHOL WITHDRAWAL

Alcohol withdrawal can be a problem both medically and behaviorally. The biggest danger is delirium tremens (DTs), which has up to a 15% mortality rate. Watch for symptoms of hyperautonomia (confusion, tachycardia, dilated pupils, and diaphoresis) usually 2 to 7 days after the last drink, although other symptoms (including seizures) can occur before then. DTs should be managed with benzodiazepines promptly. Continued supportive hydration and electrolyte maintenance are essential. If the patient is not in imminent danger but is symptomatic, consider management with the following steps until substance abuse treatment can be arranged:

- Place the patient in an environment where the patient is not endangering him- or herself or others.
- Consider lorazepam (Ativan), 0.5–1 mg PO/IV/IM q6–8h (scheduled or prn) or chlordiazepoxide (Librium), 100 mg PO q6h (up to 500 mg in the first 24 hours), for symptoms of withdrawal. Use sitter or restraints as necessary.
- A "banana bag" including thiamine, 100 mg, an IV-soluble multivitamin, and folate, 1 mg IV, should be included in all admission orders for patients with alcohol abuse. There is no magic to the IV formulation; if they can take PO, great.
- Strongly encourage the patient to seek substance abuse treatment and counseling. Social workers can assist with suggestions, and chemical dependency consultation can also be arranged for inpatient and outpatient detoxification. See also the Chemical Dependency section in Chapter 17.

BLEEDING AT LINE SITES AND AFTER PROCEDURES

Bleeding at central line sites is a common problem. Consider coagulation disorders and antiplatelet and anticoagulation drugs as causes of bleeding. Confirm that the bleeding does not extend into the soft tissues of the neck, causing upper airway obstruction. If so, an emergent ENT consult should be called. Otherwise, consider the following steps:

• Under sterile conditions, remove the dressing and apply continuous pressure (no peeking!) to the entry site for 15 minutes. If the bleeding has stopped, clean the site and apply occlusive dressing. A 4 × 4 gauze pad (or stack of two or three) folded into quarters and taped down snugly helps hold pressure after you have finished. If bleeding has not stopped, suspect a coagulation disorder. A single suture may help provide hemostasis if a small subcutaneous vessel was punctured.

• When bleeding occurs after cardiac catheterization, the cardiology fellow should be notified immediately. Initial management can be occlusive pressure dressing and sandbag. Consider obtaining a CBC and a noncontrast abdominal CT to evaluate for a retroperitoneal hematoma if there is protracted bleeding or hemodynamic compromise.

CONSTIPATION

Constipation is one of the most common complaints or calls of hospitalized patients and is something you can usually handle over the telephone. Make sure the patient isn't having N/V, abdominal pain, or fecal impaction. If these are suspected, you must see the patient. Otherwise, consider the following agents:

• Docusate (Colace), 100 mg PO bid (stool softener). Consider giving as prevention to any patient on narcotics or bedridden patients. Usually it doesn't produce the necessary effect desired unless used prophylactically (any new narcotic order should include some kind of PRN bowel regimen).

• Senna (Senokot), two tablets PO up to four times a day prn or senna/docusate (Senna-S), two tablets PO bid prn.

• Bisacodyl (Dulcolax), 10 mg PO/PR prn (stimulant).

• Consider enemas if oral agents have not been effective. Fleets or tap water enemas can be used. Do not order enemas in a neutropenic patient. Never give a patient in renal failure a phosphosoda enema.

If the above don't work, consider:

• Lactulose, 30 cc PO q4–6h until bowel movement (beware of bloating, especially in a patient with an ileus—never use until obstruction ruled out).

• Polyethylene glycol (Miralax), 17 g dissolved in 4–8 oz H_2O PO q day.

• Magnesium citrate 150–300 mL PO q day-bid.

COUGH

Cough is one of the most irritating symptoms both for the patient and the house officer. Make sure the patient isn't having massive hemoptysis (defined as >600 mL over 48 hours or enough to impair gas exchange) and try to diagnose the underlying cause. Symptomatically, consider the following steps:

- Guaifenesin/dextromethorphan or codeine (Robitussin DM or AC), 10 mL PO q4h prn
- Codeine, 10–20 mg PO q4–6h prn.
- Benzonatate capsules (Tessalon Perles), 100 mg PO tid.

DIARRHEA

Diarrhea is defined as increasing frequency and/or increasing fluidity of stools. Acute diarrhea is frequently self-limited. Determine the extent of associated symptoms (N/V, blood in stools, abdominal pain). Don't forget the possibility of ischemic colitis and fecal impaction with overflow incontinence. Be careful about patients on corticosteroids with minimal abdominal symptoms having an intra-abdominal process.
  Consider the following items:

- NPO with IV hydration.
- Correct electrolytes.
- Discontinue possible causes including laxatives, antibiotics, antacids with magnesium.
- Check CBC, stool samples (for WBC, culture and sensitivity, ova and parasites), and *C. difficile* toxin if indicated.
- Loperamide, 4 mg initially, and then 2 mg PO with each loose bowel movement. Be cautious with infectious colitis.
- Bismuth subsalicylate (Pepto-Bismol), 30 mL PO q6h.

FALLS

This is a call where you must go see the patient. Find out from the patient what occurred and where he or she is having pain. Talk with witnesses. Ask nursing for a bedside glucose test and vital signs. Examine the patient, including a careful musculoskeletal and neurologic exam, and look for any signs of injury. Clearly document what occurred in the patient's chart.

Other steps to consider include the following:

- If you have any concerns about head trauma or note a change in mental status or the patient is on anticoagulants or has a coagulopathy, check a STAT head CT without contrast to rule out a bleed. Check plain films if skeletal injury is suspected.
- Check recent lab results and ECG/telemetry. Consider checking films for possible trauma.
- Look at the medication list for possible contributing factors (sedatives, antihypertensives, hypoglycemic agents).
- Place patient on fall precautions. Consider q2h neurological checks by nursing for the next 12–24 hours in patients with head injuries.

HYPERGLYCEMIA AND HYPOGLYCEMIA

Hyperglycemia

The severity should be determined by the glucose level and the patient's symptoms. Confirm that the patient is not receiving IV fluids containing glucose. Most type 2 diabetics should be on a scheduled sliding scale insulin dose. A conservative scale is as follows, with Accu-Chek qid:

Glucose	Regular Insulin Subcutaneously
60–200	0 units
201–250	2 units
251–300	4 units
301–350	6 units
351–400	8 units
>400	10 units and call house officer
<60	1 Amp D50 IV and call house officer. If taking PO, can give PO juice/crackers, etc.

- Severe hyperglycemia with DKA is a medical emergency and is not covered here.
- All type 1 diabetics require scheduled dosages of insulin, even if they are NPO. Give 1/2 to 2/3 of usual basal insulin dose to patients who are NPO. If patient will be NPO >24 hours, consider starting IV insulin and IV glucose drips and titrate to keep blood glucose between 100 and 200.

Hypoglycemia

Any symptomatic patient with hypoglycemia should be treated.

- For mild hypoglycemia in an awake patient, oral sweetened juices can be given.
- With increasing severity, or if the patient is not able to take PO, D50 should be given IV (1 Amp).
- If IV access is unavailable with severe hypoglycemia, glucagon, 1 mg SC or IM, can be given.
- Review the patient's medications for any that may cause hypoglycemia (oral hypoglycemics, quinine, sulfa drugs).
- If ongoing hypoglycemia occurs or the patient is NPO, start a maintenance D5W infusion at 75–100 mL/hr.

HOLDING MEDICATIONS FOR MORNING TESTS

Many tests require that patients are NPO. Always consider making patients NPO after midnight if there is potential for testing the following day. Most orders are written NPO after midnight except medications. Certain tests (cardiac stress tests) require that you also hold β-blockers and calcium channel blockers the morning of the test. Hold metformin (Glucophage) 24 hours prior to studies involving IV iodinated contrast. If the test is canceled, make sure to restart the diet. For specific recommendations, please refer to Preparation for Radiologic and Endoscopic Procedures in Chapter 16.

INSOMNIA

Insomnia is a common problem in the hospital. The patient's mental status must be considered before administering medications. Make sure delirium and dementia aren't present as well as pain that may be keeping the patient awake.

Otherwise, consider use of the following agents:

- Antihistamines such as diphenhydramine (Benadryl), 25 mg PO before sleep prn. Be conscious of anticholinergic side effects, especially in the elderly.
- Zolpidem (Ambien) or zaleplon (Sonata), 5–10 mg PO before sleep prn.
- Benzodiazepines, such as temazepam (Restoril), 15–30 mg PO before sleep prn.
- Ramelteon (Rozerem), 8 mg PO before sleep prn.

LACK OF INTRAVENOUS ACCESS

Determine if IV access is necessary (i.e., essential IV medications such as antibiotics, transfusions, etc.). Consider if IV medications can be given orally.

If access is necessary, see the patient and attempt peripheral line placement. If not successful, consider other types of access such as PICC lines. If these are not options, consider central venous access. Please refer to Guide to Procedures in Chapter 18.

NAUSEA AND VOMITING

Nausea and vomiting are always symptoms of an underlying etiology (like having eaten hospital food on- or postcall). While working up the underlying cause and eliminating life-threatening etiologies, consider using the following agents:

- Prochlorperazine (Compazine), 5–10 mg IV/PO/IM q4–6h prn (also in suppository form, 25 mg bid).
- Promethazine (Phenergan), 25 mg PO/IM/PR q4–6h prn.
- Metoclopramide (Reglan), 10 mg PO/IV/IM q6h prn.
- Ondansetron (Zofran), 4–8 mg PO/IV q8h prn (for refractory cases).

PRURITUS

While identifying the underlying cause, consider the use of the following agents:

- Diphenhydramine (Benadryl), 25–50 mg PO q6–8h prn or nonsedating antihistamine such as fexofenadine (Allegra), 180 mg PO q day.
- Hydroxyzine (Atarax, Vistaril), 25 mg PO q6–8h prn.
- Sarna lotion.
- For refractory pruritis, consider doxepin 5% cream q3–4h prn or doxepin 25 mg PO q day (short-term use only).

RASH

First, make sure that this is not an *anaphylactic* reaction. Specifically look for an urticarial rash with associated SOB, wheezing, laryngeal edema, and hypotension. If these symptoms are present, consider the following items:

- Large-bore (16 gauge) access for IV fluids.
- Epinephrine, 0.5 mg (1:1,000 solution) IV or subcut.
- Diphenhydramine (Benadryl), 50 mg IV or 50–100 mg IM.
- Hydrocortisone, 500 mg IV or methylprednisolone 125 mg IV.
- Albuterol 2.5 mg by nebulizer can be administered for bronchospasm.
- Intubation if the airway is compromised.

The most common cause of rashes in-house is a *drug reaction.* Hold medication that may be the cause if this is not an essential medication. Consider a dermatology or allergy consult (for desensitization) in the AM if the medication is necessary. For symptomatic relief:

- Diphenhydramine (Benadryl), 25–50 mg PO q6–8h prn; hydroxyzine (Atarax), 25 mg PO q6–8h prn; fexofenadine (Allegra), 180 mg PO q day; or loratadine (Claritin), 10 mg PO q day if itching is present.
- Corticosteroid creams.
- Consider PO steroids such as prednisone, if severe.

SUNDOWNING

This is a common call overnight. Risk factors for sundowning include increased age, dementia, and ICU admission. The patient can present with confusion, disorientation, or combativeness in the evening hours. Things to consider:

- Identify and treat any underlying conditions that could be contributing.
- Minimize sedation. If absolutely necessary, haloperidol (Haldol), 0.25 mg PO/IM q day; risperidone (Risperdal) 0.5 mg PO qpm; or olanzapine (Zyprexa), 5 mg; for all of these, increase as needed.
- Maintain a quiet structured environment to help calm the patient down. Provide frequent reorientation; family members can be helpful in this respect.
- Consider a sitter or a bed alarm if the patient wanders. Avoid restraints if possible as they can worsen agitation and confusion.

TRANSFUSION REACTIONS

If an **acute hemolytic reaction** is suspected, follow these steps:

• Immediately stop the transfusion and send bags and patient's blood sample to the laboratory for testing, including cross-match, Coombs' test, CBC, DIC panel, total bilirubin, and BMP.
• Rehydrate with intravascular fluid.
• Closely monitor renal function, electrolytes (especially K), and coags.
• Keep urine output >100 mL/hr.

If **severe, nonhemolytic reaction** is suspected (including anaphylactic symptoms, wheezing, respiratory distress, temperature >40°C):

• D/C transfusion and send bag and line for repeat cross-match.
• Consider diphenhydramine, 25–50 mg PO/IV.
• Consider hydrocortisone, 500 mg IV.
• Consider epinephrine, 0.5–1.0 mL (1:1,000) IM.

For **volume overload**:

• Decrease rate of transfusion.
• Consider furosemide, 20–40 mg IV.

For **fever <40°C or chills**:

• Slow down rate of transfusion.
• Acetaminophen, 650 mg PO.
• Meperidine 20–50 mg IV can be used for chills.
• Continue monitoring.

Pain Control

14

. . . As if anything could control your pain . . .

GENERAL POINTS

- Treating undiagnosed pain can be perilous; always have a plan under way to diagnose the source and type of pain you are treating.
- Pain is often an undertreated symptom; once a diagnosis is made, the patient should have enough pain medications to keep him or her comfortable.
- Scheduled pain medications at appropriate doses are a viable alternative to try before switching or adding medications.
- Long-acting pain medications can improve compliance and reduce some side effects.
- *Avoid IM injections.* Subcutaneous opioids are equally efficacious and less painful than IM injections.
- Standing pain medication orders (e.g., "patient can refuse" or "for breakthrough pain") can minimize phone calls and interrupted sleep. You will want to be notified if the patient's pain or symptoms(s) persist or worsen as this may signal a change in the patient's condition.
- Consider getting an anesthesia or pain consult for other options in persistent, severe, uncontrolled pain.
- Before prescribing pain medications, always consider comorbidities, allergies, drug interactions, and potential side effects.
- Select alternative agents to meperidine, propoxyphene, and codeine (for pain) to limit potential side effects and drug interactions.
- Trust your instincts. If you think a patient is manipulative and drug-seeking, set your boundaries and stick with them. Questions to ask:
  - Does the patient only ask for pain medications when you are in the room?
  - Do others observe different behaviors when you leave the room?

- Is the patient talking or resting comfortably?
- Is the patient allergic to every pain medication except the one he or she is requesting?

Equipotent Analgesic Doses of Opioids (Tables 14.1 and14.2)

Equipotent analgesic doses are approximate, and clinical conversions should be done carefully.

1. Calculate the total opioid dose used in the previous 24 hours.
2. Convert the total dose to an oral morphine equivalent using Table 14.2.
3. Convert from oral morphine equivalent to the new opioid.
4. Give 50% of the calculated daily dose to account for incomplete cross-tolerance between opioids.

TABLE 14-1	EQUIPOTENT OPIOID DOSES			
Drug (trade name)	SQ/IV Dose (mg)	PO Dose (mg)	Duration (hours)	Half-life (hours)
Short half-life opioids				
Morphine (many)	10	30	4	2–3.5
Oxycodone (various)	—	30	4	3
Hydromorphone (Dilaudid)	1.5	7.5	4	2–3
Hydrocodone (various)	—	30	4	3–4
Fentanyl	0.1	—	1–2	1.5–6
Long-acting opioids				
Methadone (various)	10	20	6–12	15–>100

Note: Duration of analgesic effect is for single dose administration. To achieve steady state, it takes five half-lives. Exert caution when starting long half-life opioids.

Adapted from Barnes-Jewish Hospital Department of Pharmacy. Washington University Medical Center, St Louis, 2007.

TABLE 14-2	SELECTED AGENTS IN THE THREE-STEP ANALGESIC LADDER	

Agent	Oral	Parenteral
Step 1. Mild pain: nonopioid (± adjuvant)		
Acetaminophen	650 mg q4–6h PRN or 1,000 mg q6h prn	—
Aspirin	650 mg q4–6h PRN or 1,000 mg q6h prn	—
Ibuprofen	400–800 mg q6–8h prn	—
Gabapentin (for neuropathic pain)	Start 300 mg qhs	—
Step 2. Moderate pain: opioid formulated for mild/mod pain (± nonopioid; ± adjuvant)		
Hydrocodone 5 mg/acteminophen 325 mg	1–2 tablets PO q4–6h prn	—
Oxycodone 5 mg/acetaminophen 325 mg	1–2 tablets PO q4h prn	—
Oxycodone	5 mg q4–6h	—
Tramadol	50–100 mg q4–6h (maximum, 400 mg/day)	—
Step 3. Severe pain: opioid formulated for mod/severe pain (± nonopioid; ± adjuvant)		
Morphine	10–30 mg q3–4h (around the clock or in- termittent dosing)	0.1–0.2 mg/kg (up to 15 mg) q4h
Morphine (controlled release)	Can start 30 mg q8–12h and increase PRN to 90–120 mg q12h	—
Fentanyl[a]	—	0.1 mg q1–3h
Hydromorphone	2–4 mg q4–6h	1–4 mg q4–6h
Levorphanol	2 mg q6–8h	2 mg q6–8h

[a]Transdermal fentanyl: 100 µg/hr = 315–404 mg/day of oral morphine and 53–67 mg/day of IM morphine.

Adapted from Jacox et al., 1994; and World Health Organization, 1996.

5. Schedule the dosing frequency based on the analgesic half-life (e.g., for morphine: q4h; ms Contin: q8–12h; oxycodone: q4h, OxyContin: q12h).

6. Divide the calculated 24-hour dosage by the number of doses to be given daily.

7. Add PRN doses of the new opioid (short-acting form) at 5%–15% of the total daily dose for breakthrough pain.

Therapeutic Considerations

15

. . . Dose, trough, peak—just a therapeutic level I seek . . .

Antibiotics and anticoagulation are two of the most common therapeutics in the hospital setting.

ANTIBIOTICS

General Points

Three main issues must be addressed when selecting antibiotics:

1. Expected pathogen and patient demographics (i.e., nosocomial, immunocompromised).
2. Patient allergies.
3. Renal and hepatic function.

See *The Sanford Guide to Antimicrobial Therapy* for specific choices by site as well as renal dose adjustments and drug interactions.

Some Specifics on Commonly Used Antibiotics

Vancomycin

Use in severe Gram-positive infections or MRSA/ORSA. The dose is based on body weight, whereas the dosing interval is based on creatinine clearance.

Body weight (kg)	Dose (mg)
<45	500
45–60	750
61–90	1,000
>90	1,250–1,500

CRCL (mL/MIN)	Interval
>60	12 hr
35–60	24 hr
15–34	48 hr
<15	Random dosing

- Drug levels are not recommended for patients receiving a short course of therapy (<5 days).

- Periodic trough levels (every week) are recommended in patients receiving longer courses of therapy to ensure concentrations are adequate. Trough levels should be obtained approximately 30 minutes before the next dose. Therapeutic trough levels range from 5–15 mg/mL for mild to moderate infections and from 15–25 mg/mL for more severe infections. Peak levels are generally not of benefit. Hemodialysis patients should have a serum drug level measured every 4–7 days to determine timing of subsequent doses.
- Serum creatinine should be monitored weekly.

Aminoglycosides

Aminoglycosides are active against aerobic Gram-negative bacteria. Synergistic with β-lactam antibiotics. Adverse effects include ototoxicity, nephrotoxicity, and neuromuscular paralysis.

Extended interval (i.e., infrequent dosing) regimens are generally recommended. Exceptions include pregnancy, dialysis, CrCl <20, and endocarditis, where traditional-based dosing is recommended.

Extended Interval Aminoglycoside Nomogram (Fig. 15-1)

- Initial dose:

  Gentamicin, 5 mg/kg (round to nearest 50 mg)

  Tobramycin, 5 mg/kg (round to nearest 50 mg)

  Amikacin, 15 mg/kg (round to nearest 100 mg)

- Use IBW to calculate dose.

  For men: IBW = 50 kg + 2.3 (height [inches] − 60)

  For women: IBW = 45.5 kg + 2.3 (height [inches] − 60)

  If >20% above IBW, use formula IBW + 0.4 (actual body weight − IBW)

CRCL (mL/MIN)	Interval
>60	24 hr
40–59	36 hr
20–39	48 hr
<20	Use traditional dosing

- Obtain midinterval drug level 8–12 hours after the initial dose, then evaluate based on nomogram.
- Repeat drug level 1–2 times weekly and monitor serum creatinine 2–3 times weekly (Fig. 15-1).

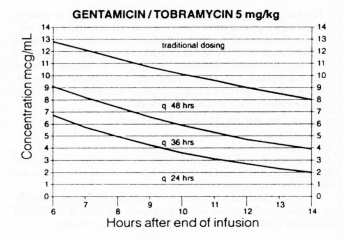

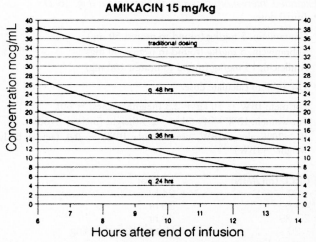

Figure 15-1 Extended interval aminoglycoside nomogram. (From Barnes-Jewish Hospital Department of Pharmacy. St. Louis: Washington University Medical Center, 2007.)

Traditional Aminoglycoside Dosing
Loading Dose

- Gentamicin, tobramycin

  For urinary tract infection or synergy against Gram-positive cocci (GPC): 1–1.5 mg/kg

  For systemic illness: 2 mg/kg

  For critical illness/sepsis 2.5 mg/kg

- Amikacin

  5–7.5 mg/kg dose based on levels

Maintenance doses: See Figure 15-2. Check aminoglycoside trough immediately before third dose and aminoglycoside peak 1 hour after start of third infusion. Peaks should be 3–5 μg/mL (UTI, synergy against GPC) or 6–10 μg/mL (systemic or critical illness). Troughs should be <2 μg/mL.

Maintenance dose is a PERCENTAGE of the selected loading dose. Example: 70 kg pt with CrCl=60mL/min and pneumonia. LD=140mg, MD=120mg q12h.

CrCl (mL/min)	t1/2 (hr)	q8h	q12h	q24h
>90	3.1	84%	100%	-
80	3.4	80%	91%	-
70	3.9	76%	88%	-
60	4.5	-	84%	-
50	5.3	-	79%	-
40	6.5	-	-	92%
30	8.4	-	-	86%
25	9.9	-	-	81%
20	11.9	-	-	75%

For CrCl < 20 mL/min, give loading dose, then follow levels and redose when level drops below 2mcg/mL.

Figure 15-2 Traditional nomogram. (From Barnes-Jewish Hospital Department of Pharmacy. St. Louis: Washington University Medical Center, 2007.)

ANTICOAGULATION

> *. . . No bleed should be your creed . . .*

Before initiating anticoagulant therapy, ensure that the patient has no history of active peptic ulcers, recent stroke or bleeding, or recent surgery. All patients should have a digital rectal examination and documented guaiac status.

Heparin Weight-Based Dosing (Unfractionated)

• Initial bolus—round to the nearest 100 units.

Acute MI: 60 units/kg, maximum 4,000 units.
DVT/PE: 80 units/kg, no maximum.
Non-DVT/PE or acute MI: 60 units/kg, maximum of 5,000 units.
High risk of bleeding: Consider smaller bolus.

• IV infusion rate.

Acute MI: 12 units/kg/hr, maximum 1,000 units/hr.
DVT/PE: 18 units/kg/hr.
Non-DVT/PE or acute MI: 14 units/kg/hr.
High risk of bleeding: 12 units/kg/hr.

An activated PTT should be ordered 6 hours after initial bolus and 6 hours after each rate change. After two consecutive aPTTs are therapeutic (60–94 sec), the aPTT should be monitored each morning. In addition, CBC with platelets should be monitored every 48 hours while on IV heparin.

HEPARIN NOMOGRAM

aPTT (SEC)*	Bolus	Infusion rate
<40	3,000 units	Increase by 3 units/kg/hr
40–50	2,000 units	Increase by 2 units/kg/hr
51–59	None	Increase by 1 unit/kg/hr
60–94	None	No change
95–104	None	Decrease by 1 unit/kg/hr
105–114	Hold for 30 min	Decrease by 2 units/kg/hr
>114	Hold for 1 hr	Decrease by 3 units/kg/hr

*Activated partial thromboplastin time (aPTT) can vary depending on lab; check local scale.

Low-Molecular-Weight Heparin Dosing

- **Enoxaparin:** 1 mg/kg subcutaneously (SC) q12h (unstable angina or DVT). If CrCl 10–30 mL/min use 1 mg/kg SC q24h (DVT/PE). Avoid use it CrCl <10 ml/minor on hemodialysis.
- **Dalteparin:** 120 units/kg SC q12h (unstable angina) or 200 units/kg subcutaneously q12h (DVT).
- **Fondaparinux** (synthetic selective Factor Xa inhibitor): 7.5 mg SC qd (DVT/PE); use 5 mg SC qd if wt <50 kg, 10 mg SC qd if wt >100kg.
- Dosages need to be adjusted in patients with renal failure. Only unfractionated heparin is recommended for patients with a CrCl

WARFARIN NOMOGRAM (FOR STARTING WARFARIN THERAPY)

Day	INR	Dosage (mg)
1	—	5
2	<1.5	5
	1.5–1.9	2.5
	2–2.5	1–2.5
	>2.5	0
3	<1.5	5–10
	1.5–1.9	2.5–5
	2–3	0–2.5
	>3	0
4	<1.5	10
	1.5–1.9	5
	2–3	0–3
	>3	0
5	<1.5	10
	1.5–1.9	7.5–10
	2–3	0–5
	>3	0

Note: Warfarin affects the CYP450 system and therefore has numerous drug interactions; consider monitoring levels of drugs metabolized by the CYP450 system while patient is on warfarin. Assistance with warfarin initiation can be found at: www.warfarindosing.org.

From Yusen RD, Eby C, Walgren R. Disorders of hemostasis and thrombosis. In *Washington Manual of Medical Therapeutics, 32nd edition.* Lippincott Williams & Wilkins, 2007.

<10 or on hemodialysis. Antifactor Xa can be checked in patients with CrCl <30 mL/min. Risk of bleeding is increased in patients with antifactor Xa levels above 0.8 units/mL.

Guidelines for Antithrombotic Therapy
* Atrial fibrillation/atrial flutter, goal INR 2–3.
  1. For cardioversion, if rhythm has been present >48 hours, anti-coagulate for 3 weeks prior to procedure and 4 weeks afterwards.
  2. For rate-controlled patients—lifelong.
  3. For patients at low risk (no h/o CVA, TIA, HTN, DM, heart disease, age <75 years) or in patients in whom warfarin therapy is contraindicated, consider ASA 325 mg q day only.

* **DVT/PE,** goal INR 2–3.
  1. First episode—3–6 months.
  2. >1 episode—lifelong.

* **Tissue or St. Judes valve in aortic position**, goal INR 2–3.
  1. Tissue—3 months.
  2. St. Judes in aortic position—lifelong.

* **Mechanical valve** (except St. Judes in aortic position), goal INR 2.5–3.5.
  1. Mechanical—lifelong.
  2. Consider adding ASA for caged-ball or caged-disc valves, if h/o CAD, embolism, or mitral valve replacement.

Treatment of High INR
Any INR >5
Hold warfarin. Search for occult bleed. Evaluate for food or drug inter-actions and dosing errors, follow INR.

INR 5–9 without Bleeding
Hold warfarin and monitor INR; can also administer vitamin K_1, 1–2.5 mg PO if at increased risk of bleeding or patient requires urgent surgery. Document decrease in INR within 48 hours. Give additional vitamin K_1 if INR remains high.

INR >9 without Bleeding
Hold warfarin; give vitamin K_1 3–10 mg PO or IVPB; follow INR every 8 hours, and repeat vitamin K_1 as needed. Consider admitting the patient if close follow-up is not possible.

Minor Bleeding
Hold warfarin; give vitamin K_1, 1–5 mg PO or IVPB; follow INR every 8 hours, and repeat vitamin K_1 as needed. If bleeding not controlled, treat as for major bleeding.

Major Bleeding
Hold warfarin; admit patient; give vitamin K_1 10 mg IVPB over 20 min, Give FFP and/or Factor VII concentrate (rFVIIa); follow INR every 6 hours; and repeat vitamin K_1 and FFP or rFVIIa q12h until INR <1.3 and bleeding has stopped. Control bleeding as needed through transfusions, surgery, etc.

Notes
Vitamin K_1 can be given in equivalent dosages PO, subcutaneously, or IVPB. Oral administration is preferred for nonlife-threatening bleeding; IV administration should be reserved for major bleeding. The response to subcutaneous administration is less predictable, but it is still effective.

If vitamin K_1 is given IVPB, administer slowly to minimize risk of anaphylactoid reaction.

Tools of the Trade (Fluids, Electrolytes, Electrocardiography, Radiology)

16

FLUIDS AND BASIC ELECTROLYTES

Basal Requirements

. . . To start 'em up . . .

Water
- Basal water requirement may be calculated as follows:
  - For the first 10 kg of body weight, 4 mL/kg/hr plus,
  - For the second 10 kg of body weight, 2 mL/kg/hr plus,
  - For remaining weight above 20 kg, 1 mL/kg/hr.
- Fever, increased respiratory rate, and sweating can all increase insensible water losses. Insensible losses increase by 100–150 mL/day for each degree of body temperature above 37°C.

Electrolytes
- Sodium: 50–150 mmol/day (as NaCl). Most of this is excreted in the urine.
- Chloride: 50–150 mmol/day (as NaCl).
- Potassium: 20–60 mmol/day (as KCl), assuming renal function is normal. Most of this is excreted in the urine.

Carbohydrates
- Dextrose, 100–150 g/day.
- IV dextrose administration minimizes protein catabolism and prevents ketoacidosis.

Maintenance Intravenous Fluids

. . . To keep 'em going . . .

- Basal requirements of water, electrolytes, and carbohydrates can be conveniently administered as 0.45% NaCl in 5% dextrose plus 20 mmol/L KCl.

- Fluid losses can be divided as urinary losses and all other losses. Urinary losses for the average adult are 0.5–1 mL/kg/hr (e.g., 70 kg person produces approximately 40–60 mL/hr or 1,200 mL/day). Other losses (water lost in sweat, stool, hydration, insensible losses) total approximately 800 cc/day.
- For average sized adults, 2–3 L (90–125 mL/hr) of this IV solution per day is sufficient (i.e., $D_5$1/2 NS + 20 mEq KCl @ 100 mL/hr).
- Patients with hypovolemia require more aggressive fluid resuscitation, generally with 0.9% NaCl. Patients with renal failure or CHF may require less.
- GI and renal losses may significantly increase the loss of water, Na^+, and K^+. Serum electrolytes should be followed closely in these situations.

ELECTROLYTE ABNORMALITIES

. . . If it's high, lower it. If it's low, get it back up . . .

Hyponatremia

. . . Please pass the salt . . .

Etiology
- **Hypotonic hyponatremia** is usually caused by primary water gain or Na^+ loss. Na^+ loss may be the result of renal or extrarenal causes.
- **Hypertonic hyponatremia** is caused by an increase in extracellular solute concentration (e.g., hyperglycemia or IV mannitol administration).
- **Isotonic hyponatremia (pseudohyponatremia)** occurs as a result of a decrease in the aqueous phase of plasma (e.g., hyperproteinemia, hyperlipidemia). The concentration of Na^+ per liter of plasma water is normal.

Evaluation
- A careful H&P should be done, paying close attention to fluid status and the neurologic examination.
- Plasma osmolality, urine osmolality, and urine Na^+ should be measured.
- Refer to Figure 16-1.

Treatment
- Mild asymptomatic hyponatremia generally requires no treatment.
- For isovolemic and hypervolemic hypotonic hyponatremia, consider fluid restriction.

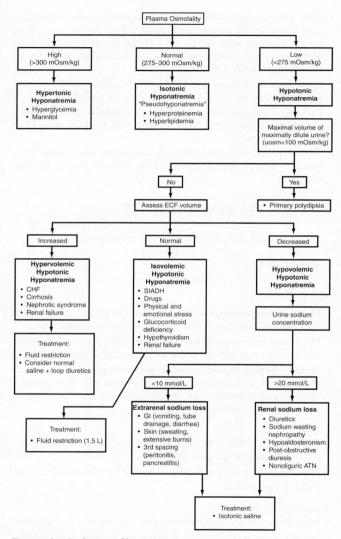

Figure 16-1 Evaluation of hyponatremia.

- For hypovolemic hypotonic hyponatremia, consider saline therapy.
- Careful consideration should be given to the rate of correction of the serum [Na$^+$]. Too rapid correction may result in osmotic demyelination or central pontine myelinolysis.
- Rapidly developing hyponatremia tends to develop with CNS symptoms and requires more rapid correction. **Severe** symptomatic hyponatremia should be treated with hypertonic saline. The rate of increase of the plasma [Na$^+$] should not exceed 1–2 mmol/L/hr with no more than 8 mmol/L in the first 24 hours.
- If acute or severe with symptoms, correct [Na$^+$] to 120–125 in first 24 hours, usually with hypertonic saline, and then gradually until completely corrected over 3–5 days.
- The quantity of [Na$^+$] required to increase the plasma [Na$^+$] by a given amount can be estimated as follows:

$$[Na^+] \text{ deficit (mmol)} = \text{desired change in } [Na^+] \times TBW$$
$$TBW = 0.6 \times \text{body weight (kg)}$$

- For example, if the desired change in [Na$^+$] is 8 mmol in a 70 kg patient, then 336 mmol of [Na$^+$] would be required (42 × 8 = 336). This would be 0.65 L hypertonic (3%) saline (336 mmol ÷ 513 mmol/L) or 2.2 L isotonic (0.9%) saline (336 mmol ÷ 154 mmol/L).

Hypernatremia

. . . Hold the salt . . .

Etiology
- Hypernatremia is caused by Na$^+$ gain or water deficit.
- **Water deficit caused by decreased intake** may be seen in patients with limited access to water (e.g., mental status alteration, intubated patients) or impaired thirst.
- **Water loss may be the result of renal or extrarenal causes.**
- Rarely, hypernatremia may result from **excess Na$^+$ intake** (e.g., hypertonic saline or NaHCO$_3$).

Evaluation
- A careful H&P should be done, paying close attention to fluid status and the neurologic examination.
- Plasma osmolality, urine osmolality, and urine [Na$^+$] should be measured.

- Solute excretion rate = urine osmolality $\times$ urine volume.
- Refer to Figure 16-2.

Treatment
- Underlying conditions should be treated (e.g., hyperglycemia, diarrhea, etc.).
- ECF volume should be restored in hypovolemic patients with isotonic saline.

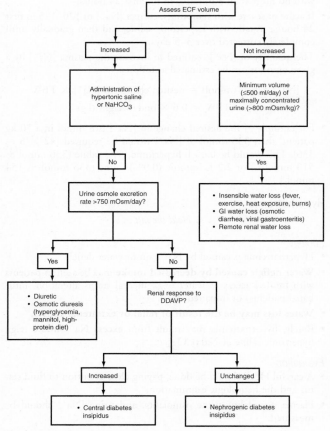

Figure 16-2 Evaluation of hypernatremia.

$$\text{Body water deficit (L)} = (\text{plasma } [Na^+] - 140)/140 \times \text{TBW (L)}$$

$$\text{TBW} = 0.6 \times \text{body weight (kg)}$$

- As with hyponatremia, too rapid correction of hypernatremia is potentially dangerous. The rate of correction of the plasma $[Na^+]$ should not exceed 0.5 mmol/L/hr and the $[Na^+]$ should decrease by no more than 12 mmol/L over the first 24 hours (or no faster than one-half of the volume deficit in the initial 24 hours).

- Don't forget to take into account ongoing losses. The safest route is PO or NG tube administration of water. Alternatively, one-half NS (0.45%), one-quarter NS (0.225%), or D5W can be given IV. Reassess volume status and Na every 8–12 hours.

- Central diabetes insipidus is treated with intranasal DDAVP.

- Nephrogenic diabetes insipidus may be reversible by treating the underlying disorder or eliminating the offending drug (e.g., lithium).

Hypokalemia

. . . More bananas, please . . .

Defined as a $[K^+]$ <3.5 mmol/L, the clinical features vary greatly. Myalgias and weakness are common complaints. Severe hypokalemia can result in an increased risk of arrhythmias. The $[K^+]$ level of cardiac patients is generally maintained above 4.

Etiology
- Hypokalemia may be caused by **decreased intake**. It is infrequently the sole cause but can exacerbate other causes of hypokalemia.

- **Intracellular shifts** (metabolic alkalosis, insulin, stress–induced catecholamine release, β–adrenergic agonists, anabolic states) may result in hypokalemia.

- K^+ depletion may also be caused by **nonrenal and renal loss**. Renal loss of K^+ may be caused by increased distal K^+ secretion or increased distal tubular flow rate. Diuretics (thiazides and loop) are a common cause. GI causes include vomiting and diarrhea. Hypomagnesemia should be ruled out.

- The transtubular potassium gradient may be useful to differentiate types of renal K^+ loss. It is calculated as follows:

$$\text{TTKG} = U[K^+]/P[K^+] \div U_{osm}/P_{osm}$$

- Calculation assumes $U_{osm} > P_{osm}$.
- TTKG <2 suggests renal loss due to increased distal flow.
- TTKG >4 suggests increased distal K^+ secretion.
- See Figure 16-3.

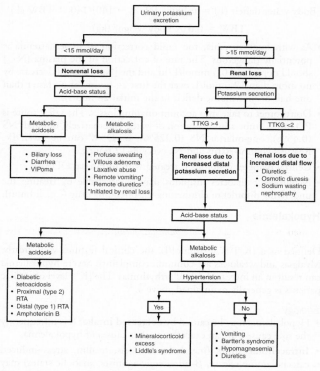

Figure 16-3 Evaluation of hypokalemia. TTKG, transtubular potassium gradient.

Evaluation
See Figure 16-3.

Treatment
- K^+ may be repleted either orally or intravenously. It is difficult to provide an algorithmic approach to replacing K^+ as the degree of depletion does not correlate well with plasma levels.
- It is generally safer and more cost effective to replace K^+ via the oral route. Caution should be used in replacing K^+ in patients with renal insufficiency. A reasonable estimate is that every 10 mEq of KCl will increase the serum level 0.05–0.1 mEq/L.

- Severe hypokalemia or patients who cannot take anything PO should be treated with IV KCl. The rate of infusion should not exceed 20 mmol/hr.
- If hypomagnesemia is present, magnesium oxide, 400 mg PO bid-tid should be given as well.

Hyperkalemia

. . . So much Kayexalate, so little time . . .

- Defined as a $[K^+]$ in excess of 5 mmol/L, the most serious effect is cardiac toxicity. If a suspicious result is received, consider repeating it STAT; a potassium can be obtained on an ABG. An ECG must be obtained. Refer to ECG interpretation section later in this chapter. Look for peaked T waves, prolonged PR interval, and QRS duration. Consider continuous cardiac monitoring if the potassium is >6.5.

Etiology
- **Pseudohyperkalemia** is caused by K^+ movement out of cells associated with venipuncture. This may be seen with repeated fist clenching, prolonged tourniquet time, hemolysis, leukocytosis, or thrombocytosis.
- **Increased K^+ intake** is an unusual cause of hyperkalemia but may be seen with excess K^+ replacement, renal insufficiency, or both.
- **Transcellular shifts** of K^+ may cause hyperkalemia. This may be seen with acidosis, insulin deficiency, drugs (succinylcholine, β-blockers), hypertonicity (e.g., hyperglycemia), hemolysis, tumor lysis, rhabdomyolysis, and hyperkalemic periodic paralysis.
- **Decreased renal K^+ excretion** is the usual cause of chronic hyperkalemia.

Major Causes of Decreased Renal Potassium Excretion
- Renal failure.
- Volume depletion.
- Primary hypoaldosteronism.
- Secondary hypoaldosteronism (e.g., diabetes, mild renal failure, chronic tubulointerstitial disease).
- Drugs (e.g., nonsteroidal antiinflammatory drugs, ACE inhibitor, angiotensin receptor blockers, heparin, spironolactone, triamterene, amiloride, trimethoprim, pentamidine).
- Tubulointerstitial disease (e.g., systemic lupus erythematosus, sickle cell disease, multiple myeloma).
- Type 4 renal tubular acidosis.

Evaluation

- Rule out pseudohyperkalemia by repeating the serum electrolytes. Consider drawing the sample without the use of a tourniquet or fist clenching.
- If the patient has thrombocytosis or marked leukocytosis, the sample may be drawn in a heparinized tube.
- Obtain a stat ECG and an ABG (if acidosis is a concern).
- Assess the patient's urine output and renal function.
- Examine the patient, paying particular attention to ECF volume status.
- Review the patient's medication list.
- Determination of plasma renin and aldosterone levels may be useful.

Treatment

- Stop all exogenous K^+ and potentially offending drugs.
- Severe hyperkalemia or hyperkalemia with ECG changes requires emergency treatment. **Do not do this by yourself.** Call your resident immediately.
- **Acute treatment:**
  - **Calcium gluconate** 10%, 10 mL IV over 2–3 minutes decreases cardiac membrane excitability. The effect occurs in minutes but lasts only 30–60 minutes. It can be repeated after 5–10 minutes if the ECG does not change. Use with extreme caution in patients receiving digoxin.
  - **Insulin**, 10–20 units IV, causes an intracellular shift of K^+ in 10–30 minutes. The effect lasts for several hours. **Glucose**, 50 g IV (1 ampule D50), should also be administered to prevent hypoglycemia.
  - **NaHCO$_3$**, 1 ampule IV can also be used to cause an intracellular shift of K^+, and the effect can last several hours. This treatment should probably be reserved for patients with severe hyperkalemia and metabolic acidosis. Patients with end–stage renal disease seldom respond and may not tolerate the Na^+ load.
  - **β_2–Adrenergic agonists** can be used to cause an intracellular shift of K^+.
  - **Diuretics** (e.g., furosemide, 40–120 mg IV) enhance K^+ excretion provided renal function is adequate.
  - **Cation exchange resins** (sodium polystyrene sulfonate, Kayexalate) enhance K^+ excretion from the GI tract. Kayexalate may be given PO (20–50 g in 100–200 mL 20% sorbitol) or as a retention enema (50 g in 200 mL 20% sorbitol). The effect

may not be evident for several hours and lasts 4–6 hours. Doses may be repeated every 4–6 hours as needed.

- **Dialysis** may be necessary for severe hyperkalemia when other measures are ineffective and for patients with renal failure.
- **Chronic treatment** is aimed at the underlying condition. Dietary K^+ should be restricted. Metabolic acidosis should be corrected. Drugs causing hyperkalemia should be avoided. Administration of exogenous mineralocorticoid may be effective for select patients.

ACID–BASE DISORDERS

. . . Retention, compensation, deficits . . .

- Changes in acid–base balance occur as a result of changes in $[H^+]$ and $[HCO_3^-]$.
- **Acidemia** results from either decreased $[HCO_3^-]$ or increased PCO_2.
- **Alkalemia** results from either increased $[HCO_3^-]$ or decreased PCO_2.
- An ABG, electrolyte panel, and a serum $[HCO_3^-]$ are required to assess acid/base status
- Stepwise approach to an ABG:
  1. Examine the pH. Is the patient acidemic or alkalemic?
  2. Examine the $[HCO_3^-]$. In primary metabolic disorders, it moves in the same direction as the pH.
  3. Examine the PCO_2. In primary respiratory disorders, it moves in the opposite direction as the pH.
  4. Is there adequate respiratory or metabolic compensation? If there is not adequate compensation, there may be a mixed disorder present (Table 16-1).
  5. If a metabolic acidosis is present, calculate the anion gap. If no gap is present, calculate the urine anion gap.

Metabolic Acidosis
Etiology
See Table 16-2.

Treatment
- Treatment of the underlying condition should be the primary focus.
- Severe acidosis (pH <7.20) may require treatment with parenteral $NaHCO_3$. Rapid infusion should be considered only for severe acidosis.

TABLE 16-1 PRIMARY ACID–BASE DISORDERS

Disorder	Abnormality	Primary Changes	Compensatory Response
Metabolic acidosis	$[HCO_3^-]$ loss or $[H^+]$ gain	$\downarrow[HCO_3^-]$	$\downarrow Pco_2$ by 1.0–1.3 mm Hg for every 1.0 mmol/L $\downarrow[HCO_3^-]$
Metabolic alkalosis	$[H^+]$ loss or $[HCO_3^-]$ gain	$\uparrow[HCO_3^-]$	$\uparrow Pco_2$ 0.6–0.7 mm Hg for every 1 mmol/L $\uparrow[HCO_3^-]$
Respiratory acidosis	Alveolar hypoventilation	$\uparrow Pco_2$	
Acute			$\uparrow[HCO_3^-]$ 1.0 mmol/L for every 10 mm Hg $\uparrow Pco_2$
Chronic			$\uparrow[HCO_3^-]$ 3.0–3.5 mmol/L for every 10 mm Hg $\uparrow Pco_2$
Respiratory alkalosis	Alveolar hyperventilation	$\downarrow Pco_2$	
Acute			$\downarrow[HCO_3^-]$ 2.0 mmol/L for every 10 mm Hg $\downarrow Pco_2$
Chronic			$\downarrow[HCO_3^-]$ 4.0–5.0 mmol/L for every 10 mm Hg $\downarrow Pco_2$

TABLE 16-2   CAUSES OF METABOLIC ACIDOSIS

Increased Anion Gap	Normal Anion Gap
Methanol	GI [HCO_3^-] loss (diarrhea, urinary diversion, small bowel, biliary, pancreatic, cholestyramine, or ingestion of Ca or Mg chloride)
Uremia	
Diabetic ketoacidosis; alcoholic ketoacidosis	
Paraldehyde	Ingestion of exogenous acids
Lactic Acidosis	Proximal (type 2) renal tubular acidosis
Ethylene glycol	Classic distal (type 1) renal tubular acidosis
Salicylates	Hyperkalemic (type 4) renal tubular acidosis
	Early renal insufficiency
	Expansion acidosis (rapid saline administration)
	Drug-induced hyperkalemia (K+-sparing diuretics, trimethoprim, pentamidine, ACE inhibitors, nonsteroidal antiinflammatory drugs, cyclosporine), carbonic anhydrase inhibitors

- The bicarbonate deficit may be calculated as follows:

$$[HCO_3^-] \text{ deficit (mEq/L)} = [0.5 \times \text{body wt (kg)}] - (24 - \text{measured } [HCO_3^-])$$

- Overaggressive correction should be avoided to prevent overshoot alkalosis.
- Hypernatremia and fluid overload can occur with $NaHCO_3$ administration.
- Serum electrolytes should be followed closely.

Metabolic Alkalosis

Etiology
- Metabolic alkalosis may be caused by HCO_3^- gain/H^+ loss or volume contraction.
- Vomiting and diuretic use are the two most common causes.
- See Table 16-3.

TABLE 16-3	CAUSES OF METABOLIC ALKALOSIS

Cl⁻ Responsive (Urine Cl⁻ <10 mmol/L)	Cl⁻ Unresponsive (Cl⁻ >10 mmol/L)
Gastrointestinal	**Normotensive**
Vomiting, NG suction	K^+ or Mg^{2+} depletion
Villous adenoma	Bartter's syndrome
Congenital chloridorrhea	Hypercalcemia
Cystic fibrosis	**Hypertensive**
Renal	Primary aldosteronism
Diuretics	Hyperreninemic
Posthypercapnic state	hyperaldosteronism
Nonreabsorbable anions (penicillin)	**Adrenal enzyme defects**
	Cushing's syndrome
Exogenous alkali (NaHCO₃⁻ massive transfusion, antacids, acetate, citrate)	Exogenous mineralocorticoid
	Pseudohyperaldosteronism (licorice, carbenoxolone,
Contraction alkalosis	tobacco chewing, Liddle's syndrome)

Treatment
- Treatment of the underlying condition should be the primary focus.
- When volume contraction is present, it should be corrected with isotonic NS.
- Hypokalemia and hypomagnesemia should be corrected.
- Cl unresponsive causes do not improve with administration of NaCl; in fact, it may be hazardous.
- K^+sparing diuretics may be effective for some forms of hyperaldosteronism.

Respiratory Acidosis
Etiology
- ↑P_{CO_2} is almost always the result of alveolar hypoventilation.
- In **acute respiratory acidosis,** the pH ↓0.08 for every 10 mm Hg ↑P_{CO_2} above 40.
- In **chronic respiratory acidosis,** the pH ↓0.03 for every 10 mm Hg ↑P_{CO_2} above 40.
- Renal compensation takes several days to develop fully.
- See Table 16-4.

TABLE 16-4   CAUSES OF RESPIRATORY ACIDOSIS

Central respiratory depression (drugs, sleep apnea, obesity, CNS disease)
Airway obstruction (foreign body, laryngospasm, severe bronchospasm)
Neuromuscular abnormalities (polio, kyphoscoliosis, myasthenia, muscular dystrophy)
Parenchymal lung disease (COPD, pneumothorax, pneumonia, pulmonary edema, interstitial lung disease)

Treatment
- Treatment is directed at the underlying condition.
- Potentially contributing drugs should be stopped or counteracted (e.g., naloxone, flumazenil).
- Ventilatory assistance may be required (CPAP or mechanical ventilation).
- Generally, $NaHCO_3$ treatment is not given unless the patient is ventilated and the pH remains severely low.

Respiratory Alkalosis

Etiology
- It is important to remember that tachypnea/hyperventilation does not necessarily imply a simple respiratory alkalosis. If you have any uncertainty, obtain an ABG.
- See Table 16-5.

TABLE 16-5   CAUSES OF RESPIRATORY ALKALOSIS

Central stimulation (anxiety, pain, hyperventilation syndrome, head trauma, CVA, tumors, fever/infection, salicylates, thyroxine, progesterone)
Hypoxemia (any causes)
Airway irritation
Decreased lung compliance (CHF, fibrosis)
Pulmonary embolism
Hepatic insufficiency/failure
Pregnancy
Hyperthyroidism
Overzealous mechanical ventilation

Treatment
- Treatment is directed at the underlying condition.
- Psychogenic hyperventilation may be treated by rebreathing from a paper bag.

ELECTROCARDIOGRAPHIC INTERPRETATION

> *. . . NSR, no abnormalities—an intern's dream . . .*

This section assumes a basic understanding of ECG reading and does not review the fundamentals.

Narrow Complex Tachycardias

Narrow complex tachycardia

Irregular rhythm	Regular rhythm
• Atrial fibrillation	• Sinus tachycardia
• Multifocal atrial tachycardia	• AV node reentrant tachycardia
	• Atrial flutter

Sinus Tachycardia
Key Features
- The P wave is of the usual morphology and rates range from 100–160 bpm.
- The QRS maintains its baseline appearance, but rate-related aberrancy occasionally occurs.
- It does not develop or resolve in a paroxysmal fashion.
- Differential diagnosis includes pain, fever, hypovolemia, hyperthyroidism, pulmonary embolism, anxiety, and ischemia.

Management
Treatment is aimed at the underlying cause.

Atrioventricular Nodal Reentrant Tachycardia
Key Features
- Probably the most common cause of paroxysmal regular SVT.
- Requires two physiologically distinct pathways of conduction (one fast and one slow) in the AV node.

- During NSR, conduction through the AV node occurs over the fast pathway.
- The rate is usually between 150 and 250 bpm.
- The QRS is usually narrow but can be widened because of a preexisting conduction delay (e.g., BBB) or rate-related aberrancy.
- In **common (typical or slow-fast) AVNRT,** there is antegrade conduction over the slow pathway and retrograde conduction back to the atria over the fast pathway, completing the reentrant circuit. Negative P waves are usually buried in the QRS but may rarely be seen in II, III, and aVF. It is usually initiated by an APC.
- In the much more **uncommon (atypical or fast–slow) AVNRT** the circuit is reversed. Negative P waves are usually seen in II, III, and aVF. It is usually initiated by a VPC.

Management
- Initial treatment of acute episodes in hemodynamically stable patients begins with vagal maneuvers (e.g., Valsalva's, carotid massage).
- If this is unsuccessful, adenosine (6 mg IV followed by 12 mg IV if necessary—halve the dosage if giving via central line) should be tried.
- Beware if there is concern for pre-excitation (shortened PR, delta waves on ECG, see Fig.16-4), as AV nodal blockade in these situations can block the normal pathway and preferentially conduct down the aberrant pathway, thus actually increasing the ventricular rate. If you're unsure, ask for help!
- Patients who are hemodynamically unstable should be electrically cardioverted.

Atrial Tachycardia
Key Features
- A single different P-wave morphology is seen in **unifocal atrial tachycardia**. Rate is usually between 100 and 200 bpm. The QRS usually maintains its baseline appearance but aberrancy can occur. It is a less common cause of SVT.

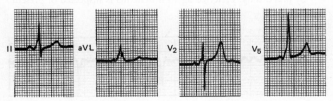

Figure 16-4 Wolff–Parkinson-White syndrome with pre-excitation.

- In **multifocal atrial tachycardia (MAT)** there are at least three separate P-wave morphologies; the rate is over 100 bpm and irregular. There is variation in the PR interval. It is most often seen in acutely ill elderly patients with pulmonary disease or CHF.

Management
- When not associated with digitalis toxicity, unifocal atrial tachycardia may be treated with calcium channel blockers or β-blockers.
- Treatment of MAT is focused on the underlying condition.

Atrial Fibrillation
Key Features
- Atrial activity is completely disorganized. The baseline is wavy without clear P waves (Fig. 16-5).
- The ventricular rate is irregularly irregular and may be slow to fast (usually >100 bpm in untreated patients).
- The QRS typically maintains its usual morphology. Variable rate-related aberrancy may also be seen.
- The incidence of AF increases with age and there are many possible causes including CAD, MI, valvular disease, PE, COPD, pericarditis, hyperthyroidism, acute alcohol intoxication, and idiopathic.

Management
- If the patient is unstable (infarction, ischemia, hypotension, mental status alteration), immediate electrical cardioversion is indicated.
- When the patient is stable, rate control may be achieved with AV nodal blocking agents:
  - Diltiazem, 0.25 mg/kg IVP over 2 minutes; if no response, repeat 0.35 mg/kg IVP over 2 minutes; follow with an IV infusion at 5–15 mg/hr. Diltiazem is probably the agent of choice in most patients. Verapamil, 5–15 mg IVP, then continuous infusion at 0.05–0.2 mg/min, can also be used.
  - Metoprolol, 5 mg IVP every 5 minutes to a total of 15 mg followed by oral dosing. Preferred agent if ischemia is suspected or present.

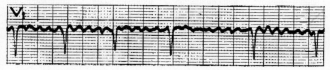

Figure 16-5 Atrial fibrillation.

- Digoxin, 0.25–0.5 mg IVP; then 0.125–0.25 mg IVP every 4–6 hours to a total dose of 0.75–1.35 mg, followed by oral dosing. Digoxin's effect will take longer than other agents.
- Amiodarone, 150 mg IV over 10 minutes, followed by infusion of 1 mg/min for 6 hours, then 0.5 mg/min for 18 hours, is not FDA approved for treatment of atrial fibrillation, but studies have shown it to be effective. Its onset of action is slower than calcium channel blockers and β-blockers. Also, be cautious if atrial fibrillation has been present >48 hours as amiodarone can cause conversion to sinus rhythm and put the patient at risk for cardioembolic stroke.
- If the patient has an EF <40% or CHF, amiodarone and digoxin are the preferred agents.
- Pharmacotherapy for AF with WPW and pre-excitation is of special concern (see previous discussion).
- In stable patients, anticoagulation is generally recommended before cardioversion (chemical or electrical) if AF has been present for >48 hours or the duration is unknown.

Atrial Flutter
Key Features
- Atrial flutter is characterized by flutter waves in a regular, undulating, sawtooth pattern at a rate of 280–350 bpm. Flutter waves are best seen in leads II, III, aVF, and V_1 (Fig. 16-6).
- The ventricular rate depends on the degree of AV block (2:1, 3:1) and may be regular or variable.
- Vagal maneuvers or adenosine may slow AV conduction, revealing the flutter waves.
- The QRS maintains its baseline appearance.
- Atrial flutter is most commonly seen in those conditions associated with AF (see previous discussion).

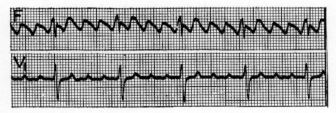

Figure 16-6 Atrial flutter.

Management
- Management of atrial flutter is similar to that for AF.
- Patients who are unstable should be immediately electrically cardioverted.
- Rate control in stable patients may be achieved in a similar manner as for AF.

Wide Complex Tachycardias

Wide complex tachycardias may be of either supraventricular or ventricular origin. Differentiation of SVT with aberrant conduction from VT on the basis of the surface ECG may be difficult (if not impossible in some patients). This differentiation is not merely academic but critical to appropriate treatment. If you find yourself in this predicament, **call for help immediately!** Regardless of the cause, if the patient is unstable (ischemia or infarction, hypotension, CHF, altered mental status), electrical cardioversion is indicated.

Ventricular Tachycardia
. . . This is bad. Really bad. Call for backup now . . .

Key Features
- VT is the most frequent life-threatening arrhythmia, and it is most often associated with MI.
- VT is defined as more than three ventricular complexes in a row at a rate of 100–250. Sustained VT lasts longer than 30 seconds or is associated with hemodynamic collapse.
- The QRS is >120 ms and often has an LBBB pattern. The T wave is usually in the opposite direction of the main QRS deflection (Fig. 16-7). It may be monomorphic (single QRS morphology) or polymorphic (multiple QRS morphologies).
- AV dissociation is present but usually cannot be easily seen.
- There may be occasional capture, fusion beats, or both.
- VT is often associated with hemodynamic compromise and has a distressing tendency to degenerate into VF and death.

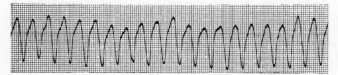

Figure 16-7 Ventricular tachycardia.

- VT can easily be confused with SVT with rate-related aberrancy or a preexistent intraventricular conduction defect, antidromic AVRT, and pre-excited AF.

Management
- If a wide complex tachycardia cannot be immediately and definitively diagnosed, it should initially be treated as VT, and you should call for help at once!
- Sustained VT (or any other wide complex tachycardia) in unstable patients requires immediate DC cardioversion by ACLS protocol.
- Pharmacologic treatment may be attempted in stable VT patients using amiodarone, lidocaine, or procainamide. **See ACLS algorithm, Chapter 2**. Of course, you'll call for help before you do this!

Torsades de Pointes
Key Features
- TDP is a rapid, polymorphic VT with QRS complexes that oscillate in amplitude and morphology, producing the appearance of a continuously twisting axis of depolarization.
- It is usually preceded by a prolonged QT interval and initiated by a VPC.
- It may be associated with electrolyte-induced long QT (most notably hypokalemia and hypomagnesemia), drugs that prolong the QT, congenital long QT syndromes, and end-stage cardiomyopathy.
- It often occurs for brief periods but can be sustained with hemodynamic collapse.

Management
- Sustained, unstable TDP should be treated with electrical cardioversion.
- Offending drugs should be stopped, and electrolyte abnormalities should be corrected.
- IV magnesium sulfate 1–2 g (up to 4–6 g) can be highly effective, even if the magnesium level is normal.

Ventricular Fibrillation
   . . . Close this book immediately! There should be multiple people running toward the patient with powerful electrical equipment . . .

Key Features
- VF is characterized by completely chaotic, rapid, highly variable amplitude electrical activity emanating from the ventricles. There are no discernible QRS complexes.

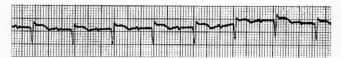

Figure 16-8 First-degree AV block.

- There is no effective cardiac output, and if VF remains untreated, it rapidly results in death.

Management
All patients require **immediate electrical cardioversion** by ACLS protocol.

Conduction Abnormalities

First-Degree Atrioventricular Block
Key Features
- The PR interval is lengthened (>200 ms), but all P waves are conducted to the ventricles (Fig. 16-8).
- It is associated with increased vagal tone, conduction system degeneration, ischemia, drugs (e.g., antiarrhythmics, calcium channel blockers, β-blockers), and electrolyte abnormalities.

Management
Primary AV block is almost always asymptomatic and rarely requires any specific treatment.

Second-Degree Atrioventricular Block, Mobitz Type I
(Wenckebach Block)
Key Features
- Not all of the atrial impulses are conducted.
- There is a progressive delay in AV conduction before a completely blocked P wave. This results in a progressive prolongation of the PR interval and shortening of the RR interval before a nonconducted P wave (Fig. 16-9).

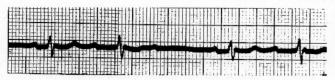

Figure 16-9 Mobitz type I (Wenckebach), second-degree AV block.

- The QRS complexes maintain their baseline appearance and appear in regular groupings. This grouping should immediately raise suspicion for Mobitz type I second-degree AV block.
- The site of conduction block is almost always within the AV node.
- Etiologies are the same as for primary AV block. Ischemia, particularly in the inferior or posterior distribution, is a common cause.
- It is usually benign and generally does not degenerate to complete heart block.

Management
- Mobitz type I second-degree AV block is usually asymptomatic and transient. Treatment is generally not necessary unless the patient is symptomatic.
- If symptomatic, atropine (0.5–1 mg IV repeated every 3–5 minutes prn to a total dose of 0.04 mg/kg) may be given, and if persistent, cardiac pacing may be necessary.

Second-Degree Atrioventricular Block, Mobitz Type II
Key Features
- Not all of the atrial impulses are conducted; however, there is no preceding conduction block.
- The PR interval is fixed and usually normal with suddenly and intermittently blocked P waves (Fig. 16-10).
- Blocked conduction may occur at a fixed ratio (e.g., 2:1, 3:1, 4:1).
- The site of conduction block is usually infranodal within the His-Purkinje system.
- Causes include increased vagal tone, conduction system disease, antiarrhythmic drugs, and ischemia (particularly in the anterior distribution).
- Mobitz type II second-degree AV block usually implies severe conduction system disease and often precedes the development of complete heart block, especially when a bundle branch block is also present. Therefore, you should always take this rhythm very seriously.

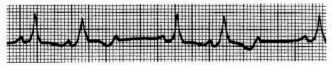

Figure 16-10 Mobitz type II, second-degree AV block.

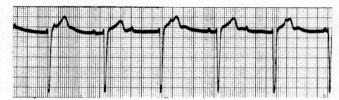

Figure 16-11 Complete heart block.

Management
- Symptomatic patients should initially be treated with atropine (0.5–1 mg IV repeated every 3–5 minutes prn to a total dose of 0.04 mg/kg), but the response is typically poor and temporary.
- Pacemaker placement is frequently indicated, regardless of whether the patient is symptomatic.

Third–Degree (Complete) Atrioventricular Block
Key Features
- As the name implies, AV block is complete, and no P waves are conducted to the ventricles (Fig. 16-11).
- An automatic focus below the block takes over at its own intrinsic rate (usually slower than the P wave rate, <50).
- There is no fixed relationship between the P waves and the QRS complexes (AV dissociation).
- The QRS complexes are usually wide but may be narrow if they arise from a junctional focus.
- The site of conduction block may be AV node or more typically within the His-Purkinje system.
- Third-degree AV block may be congenital or acquired. Etiologies of acquired complete heart block include idiopathic conduction system degeneration, ischemia or infarct, infiltrative diseases, drug toxicity, calcific aortic stenosis, endocarditis, and cardiac surgery.

Management
Emergent treatment with atropine (0.5–1 mg IV repeated every 3–5 minutes prn to a total dose of 0.04 mg/kg), and pacemaker placement is usually required.

Myocardial Ischemia and Infarction
Key Features
- Myocardial ischemia is characterized by symmetric T-wave inversion that may be slight to deep, flat or down-sloping ST depression, or both.

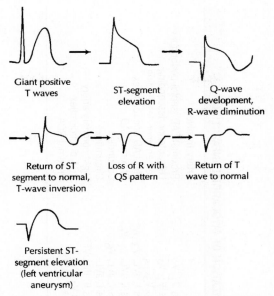

Giant positive
T waves

ST-segment
elevation

Q-wave
development,
R-wave diminution

Return of ST
segment to normal,
T-wave inversion

Loss of R with
QS pattern

Return of T
wave to normal

Persistent ST-
segment elevation
(left ventricular
aneurysm)

Figure 16-12 ST and T-wave changes in MI. (From Alpert J. *Cardiology for the Primary Care Physician.* Appleton and Lange, 1998: 168, with permission.)

- The ECG typically demonstrates sequential changes during the evolution of an acute ST-elevation MI (Fig. 16-12). Certainly not all patients show this typical sequence, and the time course of the changes may vary among patients.
- In the earliest hyperacute phase tall and prolonged T waves are seen.
- This is followed by the acute phase of convex–up ST-segment elevation in the leads facing the area of injury.
- Reciprocal ST depression may be seen in the leads opposite to the area of infarction.
- Over the following hours to days, the R-wave amplitude decreases and pathologic Q waves appear (>40 ms or greater than or equal to one-third of the entire QRS amplitude).
- As the ST segments return to baseline, the T waves become symmetrically inverted.
- Over time, the T waves may return to their baseline orientation.

TABLE 16-6 ELECTROCARDIOGRAPHIC LOCALIZATION OF MYOCARDIAL INFARCTION

Area of MI	ECG Abnormality	Artery Involved
Septal	ST elevation and Q waves V_1–V_2	Proximal LAD, septal perforators
Anteroseptal	ST elevation and Q waves V_1–V_4	Left anterior descending
Anterior	ST elevation and Q waves V_3–V_4	Left anterior descending
Anterolateral	ST elevation and Q waves I, aVL, V_3–V_6	Mid-LAD or circumflex
Extensive anterior	ST elevation and Q waves I, aVL, V_1–V_6	Proximal LAD
Lateral	ST elevation and Q waves I, aVL, V_6	Circumflex
High lateral	ST elevation and Q waves I, aVL	Circumflex
Inferior	ST elevation and Q waves II, III, aVF	Right coronary artery
Posterior	Tall R and ST depression V_1–V_2	RCA or circumflex
Right ventricular	ST elevation V_4R	Proximal RCA

- The distribution of these typical ECG changes can be used to predict the location of the myocardial infarction (Table 16-6). It is important to remember, however, that this method of localization can be rather imprecise.
- The ST segments may remain chronically elevated in the setting of LV aneurysm formation.
- Noninfarction-related Q waves can be seen in myocarditis, cardiomyopathies, muscular dystrophies, scleroderma, amyloidosis, sarcoidosis, WPW, LVH, BBB, COPD, and PE.
- Non-ST elevation MIs often have many more nonspecific and subtle ECG changes. Possible changes include persistent ST depression, T-wave inversions, loss of QRS amplitude, and poor R-wave progression across the precordium.
- Prior MIs and preexistent or newly developed conduction abnormalities may mask or make these typical changes difficult to interpret.
- Other conditions may mimic the ECG changes of an acute MI including pericarditis, myocarditis, and aortic dissection.
- It is very difficult to diagnose acute MI changes in the setting of LBBB or a paced rhythm.

Management
A detailed discussion of the management of myocardial ischemia and infarction is beyond the scope of this manual. Refer to the Chapter 12 section on chest pain for acute management and call your resident immediately.

Miscellaneous Conditions

Pericarditis
Key Features
- The acute phase of pericarditis is characterized by diffuse flat or concave–up ST–segment elevation, particularly in the precordial leads. The entire T wave may be lifted off the baseline, and there may also be diffuse PR depression (Fig. 16-13).

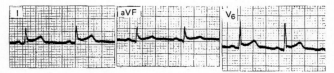

Figure 16-13 Pericarditis.

- In the intermediate phase, diffuse T-wave inversion appears and ST elevation resolves.
- In the late phase, T-wave inversion resolves.
- There is no development of Q waves.
- Pericarditis has many possible causes including infectious (viral, bacterial, fungal, tuberculous), post-MI, posttraumatic, postpericardiotomy, collagen vascular diseases, drug-induced (hydralazine, procainamide), uremia, infiltrative (sarcoidosis, amyloidosis), neoplastic, radiation, and idiopathic.

Management
- Specific, treatable causes should be managed in the appropriate manner (e.g., antimicrobial agents for infectious causes or dialysis for uremia).
- Anti-inflammatory treatment may be effective (NSAIDs or prednisone).
- Narcotic analgesics may be given for refractory pain.
- Patients should be observed closely for the development of cardiac tamponade.
- Anticoagulants should be avoided because of the risk of hemopericardium.

Hyperkalemia
Key Features
- The earliest ECG feature of hyperkalemia is tall, peaked, symmetric, narrow-based T waves. These are often referred to as "tented" T waves. They are best seen in leads II, III, and V_2-V_4 (Fig. 16-14).
- The P-wave amplitude then decreases and the PR interval becomes prolonged. With increasingly severe hyperkalemia, the P waves eventually all but disappear. Consequently, arrhythmias that are common in hyperkalemia can be difficult to identify.
- With severe hyperkalemia, the QRS progressively widens, the R amplitude decreases, and S waves become prominent. There may also be ST-segment depression or elevation.

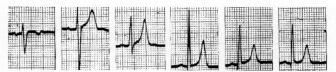

Figure 16-14 Hyperkalemia.

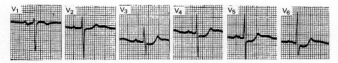

Figure 16-15 Digitalis effect.

- Eventually, with extreme hyperkalemia, the ECG takes on a slow sinusoidal pattern that may degenerate into asystole or VF if not immediately and aggressively treated.

Management
The acute management of hyperkalemia is covered in the section regarding electrolyte abnormalities earlier in this chapter.

Digitalis Effect and Toxicity
Key Features
- At therapeutic levels, digitalis may cause a characteristic, gradual down-sloping concave-up (also described as "scooping" or "sagging") of the ST segment. The ST is typically depressed and shortened and the T wave amplitude decreased. Collectively, this is known as the "dig effect" (Fig. 16-15).
- At times, it can be difficult to differentiate the dig effect from other causes of ST depression.
- Digitalis toxicity has been associated with nearly all known arrhythmias. Common digitalis toxicity-associated arrhythmias include sinus block, APCs, PAT with block, JPCs, junctional tachycardia, AV block, VPCs, VT (including bidirectional VT), and VF.
- Hypokalemia, hypomagnesemia, and hypercalcemia may enhance the toxic effects of digitalis.
- Because of its narrow therapeutic window, toxicity can occur even when the digitalis level is within the usual therapeutic range.

Management
- Digitalis should be discontinued immediately.
- In the setting of recent acute ingestion of potentially toxic amounts of digitalis and before toxic cardiac side effects have occurred, induced emesis or gastric lavage may be used. Activated charcoal may also be administered to reduce further absorption.
- The patient should be on continuous telemetry monitoring.
- Electrolyte abnormalities (particularly hypokalemia) should be carefully corrected. However, care should be taken as rapid increases in

potassium (even within the normal range) may worsen AV conduction and lead to complete heart block. Serum potassium concentration should be determined before potassium administration. Massive digitalis overdoses can cause hyperkalemia.

- Ventricular arrhythmias can be treated with IV lidocaine (1–1.5 mg/kg initial IV bolus, additional 0.5–1.5 mg/kg IV bolus injections prn up to a total of 3 mg/kg, followed by continuous IV infusion at 2–4 mg/minute), or phenytoin (250 mg IV loading dose over 10 minutes, followed by additional 100 mg IV doses every 5 minutes prn to a total of 1,000 mg). Avoid procainamide and bretylium.

- Bradyarrhythmias may be treated with atropine (0.5–1 mg IV repeated every 3–5 minutes prn to a total dose of 0.04 mg/kg) or temporary pacing.

- Digitalis-specific Fab antibody fragments (Digibind) may be given when other methods have been ineffective. One vial of Fab fragments is equivalent to 40 mg and neutralizes approximately 0.6 mg of digitalis. The dosage for chronic toxicity is calculated as follows:

    Number of vials = [dig level (ng/mL) × weight (kg)]/100

    For acute overdosages, use the following formula:

    Number of vials = [total amount ingested (mg) × 0.8]/0.5

    If acute ingestion and unknown dosage, give 10–20 vials IV. The Fab fragments are given in NS over 15–30 minutes.

- Electrical cardioversion should be used only as a last resort, when all other measures have failed. Cardioversion in the setting of digitalis toxicity can cause VT or VF that is resistant to any further cardioversion.

RADIOGRAPH INTERPRETATION

. . . Know your patients inside out . . .

Chest X-Ray

The chest x-ray is by far the most common radiograph you will order and need to interpret. When reading a chest x-ray, the most important thing is to be systematic. Be sure to check the name and date on the film and compare with old films whenever possible.

Technique
- Is the exposure correct? Underexposure can cause you to see things that aren't there, while overexposure can cause pathology to disappear. You should be able to faintly see the intervertebral spaces through the cardiac silhouette.
- Is the patient properly positioned? The spinous processes and trachea should be midline. The clavicular heads should be equidistant from the spinous processes. Rotated films distort the appearance of the cardiac silhouette and hila.
- Is the frontal film a PA or AP? AP films are often done in emergent situations or when the patient cannot stand. A two-view (PA and lateral) is optimal if the patient can tolerate it.
- Was the film taken at full inspiration? Small lung volumes can produce vascular crowding and apparent atelectasis.

Airway
- The trachea should be midline and not deviated. The trachea will deviate toward the collapsed lung (away from the side of the pneumothorax) if there is a tension pneumothorax.
- If the patient is intubated, note the position of the endotracheal tube (should be about 2 cm above the carina).

Soft Tissues
Examine the soft tissues for symmetry, subcutaneous air, edema, and breast tissue.

Bones
- Systematically look at the sternum, ribs, clavicles, spine, and shoulders.
- Look for fractures, osteolytic or osteoblastic lesions, and arthritic changes.

Diaphragm
- The sides of the diaphragm should be equal and slightly rounded. The right side may be slightly higher.
- Look for blunting of the costophrenic angles that suggest small pleural effusions.
- Flat diaphragms suggest emphysema.
- A unilateral high diaphragm may suggest paralysis, loss of lung volume on that side, or eventration/diaphragmatic tear (in the setting of trauma).

- Check for free air under the diaphragm, which is an indication of perforation.

Heart and Mediastinum

- A maximal heart width greater than half of the chest width suggests cardiomegaly or pericardial effusion.
- The aortic knob should be distinct.
- Mediastinal widening is indicative of thoracic aortic dissection or aneurysm, pericardial effusion, or mass.
- Mediastinal and tracheal deviation may be seen with pneumothorax. As above, the trachea will deviate away from the side of the pneumothorax if tension physiology is present.
- Use lateral films to confirm findings on PA and look for retrocardiac infiltrates.

Hilar Structures

- The left hilum is usually 2–3 cm higher than the right. They are generally of equal size.
- Enlarged hila suggest lymphadenopathy or enlargement of the pulmonary arteries. Use the lateral film for help in differentiating.

Lung Markings

- Look for normal lung markings all the way out to the chest wall to rule out pneumothorax. If lung markings are not seen to the periphery, look for a thin white pleural line. Be sure not to miss this! If you think you've detected a pneumothorax, let your resident know right away.
- Normal lung markings taper as they travel out to the periphery and are smaller in the upper lungs. Lung markings in the upper lung fields that are as large or larger ("cephalization") suggest pulmonary edema.
- Kerley B lines (small linear densities at the peripheral lung bases) are seen with CHF.
- Hyperlucency of the lung fields with increased retrosternal clear space on the lateral view is seen in COPD.
- Examine the lungs for the presence of infiltrates and masses.
- Obliteration of part or all of the heart border (silhouette sign) implies that the lesion/infiltrate is contiguous with or abuts the heart border. It may be located in the RML, lingula, or anterior segment of the upper lobe.

- A small pleural effusion is suggested by blunting of the costophrenic angle. Larger effusions obscure the shadow of the diaphragm and produce an upward-curving shadow along the chest wall. A straight horizontal air-fluid level indicates a concurrent pneumothorax.
- Lateral decubitus films should be done to ensure that the effusion is free flowing and large enough to attempt thoracentesis (usually >1 cm on lateral film). The side of the effusion should be down (i.e., right effusion = right lateral decubitus film).

Plain Abdominal Films

Generally speaking, plain abdominal films ("KUB" or "obstructive series") are of limited value. Despite that, they are ordered quite frequently. Again, a systematic approach is key.

Bones
- Examine the bones first lest you forget.
- Begin with the spine, then ribs, pelvis, and upper femurs. Look for signs of arthritis, fractures, and osteolytic or osteoblastic lesions.

Soft Tissues
- Systematically study the soft tissues looking for evidence of masses or calcifications. Calcifications can be seen over the gallbladder, renal shadows, ureteral course, or in the right lower quadrant (appendicolith). Phleboliths (vascular calcifications) are commonly seen in the pelvis and usually have a lucent center.
- Be sure to carefully look for free air under the diaphragm (upright film) or next to the abdominal wall (lateral decubitus film). Free air is indicative of perforation. If you see this, let your resident know immediately!

Gastrointestinal Structures
- Look for the gastric bubble. A large air-distended stomach suggests some form of obstruction.
- Observe the bowel gas pattern. A small amount of air is generally seen in the colon, while the small bowel is generally devoid of air. Fecal material is often visible in the colon although large amounts may be seen in constipation.
- The colon may become greatly distended with air in colonic obstruction (colonic distention proximal to the obstruction) or

ileus. Unless the distention is severe, the haustral markings are maintained. (The large bowel markings are differentiated from small bowel markings by their wider spacing, and the incomplete crossing of the lumen.) When the ileocecal valve is incompetent, large bowel obstruction may also cause distention of the small bowel.

- Distention of the small bowel may be seen in mechanical obstruction and ileus. Small bowel striations are much more numerous and completely cross the lumen. With mechanical obstruction there is distention proximal to the obstruction and clearing of air distally. Small bowel diameters greater than 3 cm suggest dilatation.
- The appearance of ileus is much less distinct. There is discontinuous air in the small and (usually) large bowel. The degree of distention is also less remarkable and discontinuous.
- Air-fluid levels do not distinguish mechanical obstruction from ileus. They may be seen in both conditions.

PREPARATION FOR PROCEDURES

> . . . A procedure canceled due to inadequate prep is like having a
> hemolyzed specimen. Nobody's happy, you have to do it again,
> and it's always the intern's fault . . .

General Points

- Perform plain x-ray films prior to contrast studies. Perform contrast studies prior to barium studies (i.e., start with studies that require greatest amount of clarity of the area in question). Barium can cause metallic streak artifact on CT, obscuring findings to the point it may preclude the exam until the barium is cleared from the bowel.
- Consult your radiology department if you have questions about what study to order or to confirm preparation for procedures. Some preparations are institution specific. See Table 16-7.
- Studies requiring no preparation include chest x-rays, abdominal x-rays, C-spine series, skull series, transthoracic echo, as well as those listed below.
- Remember to restart the diet postprocedure or if procedure is canceled.

Contrast Reactions

- Everyone feels a sense of warmth or flushing during contrast administration—this is not an allergy.

TABLE 16-7 PREPARATION FOR RADIOLOGY TESTS

Procedure	Preparation
CT	
Chest/extremity/head	Usually none if noncontrast, but may need contrast. If intravenous contrast is to be administered, patient should be NPO for 4–6 hr.
Abdominal/pelvic	No IV contrast needed if looking for renal stone or retroperitoneal bleed. Other types of studies usually require IV contrast if possible and may require oral depending on the patient and the indication. Discuss special protocol needs (liver, pancreas, renal protocol) and need for oral contrast with the radiologist.
MRI	None.
Ultrasound	
Abdominal	NPO starting 6 hr prior to procedure.
Pelvic	Four glasses of water 1 hr prior; no voiding 1 hr prior.
Gastrointestinal studies	
Barium swallow (used to evaluate pharynx and esophagus typically for dysphagia work–up)	NPO 4 hr prior to procedure.
Modified barium swallow (used to evaluate for possible aspiration during feeding)	NPO 1 hr prior to procedure.
Upper GI (used to evaluate the esophagus, stomach, and proximal small intestine; typically used to look for ulcers)	NPO starting midnight the day of procedure.

(continued)

TABLE 16-7   PREPARATION FOR RADIOLOGY TESTS *(Continued)*

Small bowel follow-through (contrast is followed through the small intestine; typically used to evaluate for areas of stricture or large mucosal abnormalities).	One glass of water every hour between noon and 7 PM; no smoking/chewing tobacco after midnight.
Barium enema (used to evaluate the colon for mucosal lesions such as polyps and strictures).	Clear liquids 1 day prior; NPO after midnight; 1 glass of water every hour from 1 PM to 7 PM 1 day prior, mag citrate at 8 PM, 4 Dulcolax tablets at 11 PM, 1 Dulcolax suppository at 7 AM.
HIDA scan	NPO starting midnight the day of procedure.
PET scan	NPO starting midnight the day of procedure. In diabetic patients, be sure to have the glucose under reasonable control (<300 mg/dL).
Genitourinary studies	
Cystogram	No dietary restriction full bladder.
Interventional studies	
Venogram	Clear liquids; NPO 1 hr prior to procedure.
Lymphangiogram	Light meal prior; limit fluids 2–3 hr prior to procedure. If the patient is having a procedure that will require sedation (almost all procedures other than tube or line change) the patient should be NPO 4–6 hr before the exam.
Endoscopic studies	
EGD/ERCP	NPO starting 6 hr prior to procedure.

(continued)

TABLE 16-7	PREPARATION FOR RADIOLOGY TESTS *(Continued)*
Colonoscopy	Clear liquids 1 day prior to procedure; 1 gallon of Go-LYTELY 1 cup per 15 min until done on night prior to procedure (consider NG tube if not able to complete); NPO after midnight.
Flexible sigmoidoscopy	Clear liquids starting with dinner the night before; NPO after midnight. Mag citrate at 8 PM, one glass of water every 2 hr until 10 PM, then 3 Dulcolax tablets at 10 PM, and 1 Dulcolax suppository at 6 AM.

- For known contrast sensitivity (e.g., hives, rash), consider prednisone, 50 mg PO q6h × 4 doses prior to the exam. The last dose should be administered 1 hour prior to the administration of contrast. Diphenhydramine, 50 mg PO, can also be added 1 hour prior to contrast.

- Although only nonionic contrast is used for CT (check your institution for confirmation), if your patient has had a major event with previous contrast administration (e.g., shock or airway compromise), discuss this with the radiologist **prior** to ordering a test. Patients who have had life-threatening reactions in the past should not receive IV contrast again, even with premedication. Allergic reactions generally do not occur with PO contrast.

- The contrast used in MR examinations is a gadolinium preparation, not iodinated contrast. There is cross-reactivity in some patients, so those with severe contrast reaction to CT nonionic IV contrast should receive premedication for gadolinium as well. See above for premedication regimen. In addition, there is a relationship between gadolinium administration and nephrogenic systemic sclerosis in the setting of impaired renal function. Patients with creatinine clearance <30 and hepatorenal syndromes are at high risk. Consult with your radiologist about preparatory regimens, reduction in the gadolinium load, or performing the study without contrast.

TABLE 16-8	PREPARATION FOR CARDIAC TESTS

Test	Preparation
Coronary angiogram	NPO after midnight.
Stress echo, dobutamine stress echo, or exercise stress test: 　Nuclear stress test (walking)	NPO after midnight. Hold AM doses of calcium channel blockers and β-blockers. NPO after midnight. Hold AM doses of calcium channel blockers and β-blockers.
Adenosine or dipyridamole (Persantine) nuclear stress test (nonwalking)	For diabetics on insulin only, half the normal insulin dose and eat a light meal 3 hr prior to procedure (no fats or dairy products). Avoid any xanthine-containing products (e.g., chocolate, caffeine) and theophylline or Persantine for 24 hr prior to procedure.

Contrast Nephropathy

- This is a common complication of any procedure involving iodinated IV contrast (e.g., radiological studies, angiograms). Risk factors include presence of chronic kidney disease, diabetes, and larger amount of contrast infused. Strategies for prevention include:
- IV hydration: 1 mg/kg/hr of 0.45 or 0.9 NS for 6–12 hours before and 6–12 hours after the procedure. Can also use a sodium bicarbonate solution, 3 ampules of $NaHCO_3$ (150 mEq total) in 1 L D5W. This much $NaHCO_3$ should not be put in saline due to the high sodium load.
- N-acetylcysteine (Mucomyst), 600 mg bid × 2 doses before the procedure and 2 doses after the procedure, may also be added.
- Contrast should be given cautiously to anyone with a Cr >2.0.

Gastrointestinal Radiology

- GI studies can be uncomfortable and require patient cooperation and mobility. If your patient is paralyzed, demented, angry, or delirious, the study will likely be suboptimal or may not be able to be performed.

- General rules for the "barium versus hypaque" dilemma (call the radiologist if you have specific questions):
  1. **Barium** is bad in pleural or peritoneal spaces so avoid this if perforation, obstruction, or a fistula is suspected. Do not use if the patient is likely to need a laparotomy soon.
  2. **Hypaque** is bad to aspirate, so avoid in cases of possible aspiration.

Cardiac Studies

In general:

- No smoking 2 hours prior to test, remove nicotine patches the morning of the test.
- Small sips of water with medication are fine.

MRI

- Absolute contraindications are pacemakers, ICDs, cochlear implants, and any metal in the globe and ferromagnetic intracranial aneurysm clips.
- Relative contraindications are recent operations (less than a few weeks) and recent vascular stenting. Prosthetic hip joints or metal implants are not generally contraindicated, but their artifact may obscure any adjacent lesions. If you have questions, consult MRIsafety.com or call the radiologist.
- As with CT, the patient must be able to lie still and cooperate— consider mild sedation (e.g., lorazepam) if necessary. Patients may get claustrophobic.

Ultrasound

- Abdominal ultrasounds can be used to evaluate the gallbladder, liver, and kidneys. The pancreas is typically not well visualized— use CT instead.
- Ultrasound can also locate pockets of fluid to guide paracentesis or thoracentesis.
- It is important the patient be made NPO as gas can obstruct the image.

Approach to Consultation

17

. . . With a little help from our friends . . .

THE MEDICINE CONSULT

Guiding principles for effective medicine consults were first suggested by Lee Goldman and colleagues in a paper published in the *Archives of Internal Medicine* in September 1983.

The so-called ten commandments for effective consultations are presented:

1. Determine the question being asked.
As a guiding principle, and when taking the initial phone call from the requesting service, always determine the specific medicine-related question he or she wants answered. This will be helpful, especially in situations in which the patient has an extensive and complicated previous medical history. Thus, a typical consultation note should begin by stating a specific problem, such as "Called to see this 78-year-old woman with type 2 diabetes and hypertension for perioperative glucose control. . . ."

2. Establish urgency.
Always determine if the consult is emergent, urgent, or elective.

3. Look for yourself.
Seldom do the answers to the consultation question lie in the chart; more often than not, independent data gathering is required, including reviewing prior admissions. Often the patient requires further testing. In many cases, the data review combined with a complete history and physical exam from an internal medicine perspective will establish the diagnosis.

4. Be as brief as appropriate.
It is not necessary to repeat in detail the data already in the primary team's note; obviously as much new data independently gathered should be recorded.

5. Be specific.
Try to be goal oriented and keep the discussion and differential diagnosis concise. When recommending drugs, always include dose, frequency, and route.

6. Provide contingency plans.

Try to anticipate potential problems (e.g., if using escalating doses of a β-blocker for rapid atrial fibrillation, make sure that regular BP checks are instituted). Staff (nursing/ancillary) on other floors are not used to treating medicine patients.

7. Honor thy turf.

Remember to answer the questions you were asked; it is not appropriate to engage the patient in a detailed discussion of whether surgery is indicated or likely to succeed. In situations in which you are asked by the patient about the surgical procedure, defer to the primary team rather than speculating on the technical aspects of the surgery.

8. Teach—with tact.

Share your insights and expertise without condescension.

9. Talk is cheap, and effective.

Communicate your recommendations directly to the requesting physician. There is no substitute for direct personal contact. Next month the shoe may be on the other foot, and the same resident may be coming to evaluate a surgical abdomen on one of your medicine admissions.

10. Follow up.

Suggestions are more likely to be translated into orders when the consultant continues to follow up.

Preoperative Cardiovascular Risk Assessment

- Preoperative evaluation and intraoperative management are aimed at eliminating or treating risk factors to reduce the risk of cardiac events (MI, unstable angina, CHF, arrhythmia, and death).
- Risk assessment guidelines have been published by the American College of Cardiology/American Heart Association Task Force (*Circulation* 2007;116:1971 or www.acc.org). History, physical examination, and ECG are important components of a thorough clinical assessment and help determine the extent of diagnostic testing required.
- Patients who have mild CAD on cardiac cath or successful revascularization and have no new clinical symptoms probably have a similar risk for events as patients without CAD.
- The American College of Cardiology/American Heart Association algorithm for preoperative cardiac risk assessment is detailed in Figure 17-1.
- **β-Adrenergic antagonists** should be considered in all patients with substantial risk of cardiac disease to reduce mortality and the

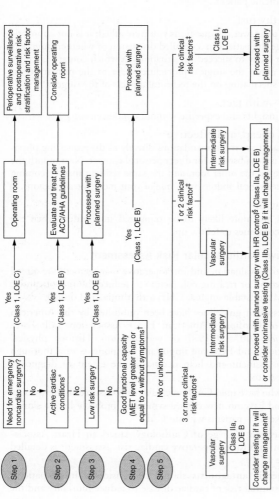

Figure 17-1 *ACC/AHA 2007 Guidelines on Perioperative Cardiovascular Evaluation and Care for Noncardiac Surgery: Executive Summary.* (From Fleisher LA, Beckman JA, Brown KA, et al. A Report of the American College of Cardiology/American Heart Association Task Force on Practice Guidelines [Writing Committee to Revise the 2002 Guidelines on Perioperative Cardiovascular Evaluation for Noncardiac Surgery]. With permission.) *Unstable coronary syndromes, decompensated CHF, significant arrhythmias, and severe valvular disease. †Walking at 4 mph on level ground, climbing stairs, climbing hills, riding a bicycle at 8 mph, golfing, bowling, throwing a baseball/football, carrying 25 lbs (groceries from the store to the car), scrubbing the floor, raking leaves, mowing the lawn. ‡Stable CAD, compensated or prior CHF, DM, CKD, and cerebrovascular disease. §Consider perioperative beta blockade. LOE, level of evidence; MET, metabolic equivalent.

Step 1

Step 2

Step 3

Step 4

Step 5

Need for emergency noncardiac surgery?

Yes (Class 1, LOE C) → Operating room → Perioperative surveillance and postoperative risk stratification and risk factor management

No

Active cardiac conditions*

Yes (Class 1, LOE B) → Evaluate and treat per ACC/AHA guidelines → Consider operating room

No

Low risk surgery

Yes (Class 1, LOE B) → Processed with planned surgery

No

Good functional capacity (MET level greater than or equal to 4 without symptoms†)

Yes (Class 1, LOE B) → Proceed with planned surgery

No or unknown

3 or more clinical risk factors‡

1 or 2 clinical risk factors‡

No clinical risk factors‡

Vascular surgery

Class IIa, LOE B

Intermediate risk surgery

Vascular surgery

Intermediate risk surgery

Consider testing if it will change management§

Proceed with planned surgery with HR control§ (Class IIa, LOE B) or consider noninvasive testing (Class IIb, LOE B) if it will change management

Class I, LOE B → Proceed with planned surgery

126

incidence of cardiovascular complications, though this has recently become somewhat controversial. For now, treatment of high risk patients seems reasonable. Lowering the HR to 50–60 bpm has been the target in most studies. If the patient is already taking a β-blocker, it should be continued and titrated to a goal HR of 50–60 beats per minute.

- Angiotensin-converting enzyme inhibitors should be considered for patients with systolic heart failure.
- Patients taking calcium channel blockers should continue this medication throughout the perioperative period.
- Continuation of preoperative antihypertensive treatment throughout the perioperative period is critical, particularly if the patient is on clonidine (risk of rebound hypertension). Consider switching the patient to IV or transdermal formulations of medications if the patient will be NPO for an extended period of time.

DERMATOLOGY

Toxic Epidermal Necrolysis (TEN)

A. *Emergency—call a consult immediately!* TEN is the most severe variant of a disease spectrum that consists of bullous erythema multiforme (EM) and Stevens-Johnson syndrome (SJS).

B. Pertinent information: drug history. Drugs are nearly always the cause, typically occurring within the first 8 weeks of therapy. The most common offenders are sulfonamides, anticonvulsants, penicillin, NSAIDs, antiretroviral medications, and allopurinol. Fewer than 5% of patients report no history of medication use.

C. Typical symptoms: begins with a prodrome of high fever, cough, sore throat, burning eyes, and malaise, 1–3 days before the onset of skin involvement.

D. Physical exam findings: high fever, painful erythema of skin, lesions rapidly coalesce producing large blisters, mucosal erosions, and conjunctival erythema. The skin eruption is usually *painful*, a key to making the diagnosis.

E. Work-up: CBC, CMP, CXR (in setting of respiratory distress), skin biopsy.

F. Diagnosis: physical exam findings and skin biopsy.

G. Treatment:
   1. Stop suspect drug(s).
   2. Transfer to burn unit/ICU.

    3. IV fluids, NG tube.

    4. Sterile protocol, antiseptic solution, and nonadherent dressings (Silvadene).

    5. Antibiotics only if highly suspicious of sepsis.

    6. Consider IVIG.

    7. Use of systemic steroids is controversial. There is no convincing evidence that steroid therapy is helpful.

    8. Ophthalmology consult.

    9. OB/GYN consult for vaginal involvement; urology consult for urethral involvement.

H. Clinical pearls: Hepatitis occurs in 10%. Most patients have anemia and lymphopenia. Neutropenia is associated with a poor prognosis. A severe drop in temperature is more indicative of sepsis than fever. Mortality ranges from 30% to 40% and is most often secondary to sepsis, renal failure due to hypovolemic shock, or ARDS. Patients with HIV, systemic lupus, or a bone marrow transplant have a higher risk of developing TEN. Stevens-Johnson syndrome is also drug induced and presents with mucosal lesions and less skin involvement. Progression of painful erythema/bullae beyond 10% to 30% of the skin may indicate a transition from SJS to TEN.

I. Prognosis: TEN has a mortality rate of 30% to 40%.

    1. SCORTEN severity of illness score (*J Invest Dermatol 2006; 126:272*):

- Age >40 years
- Heart rate >120 beats per minute
- Malignancy
- Involved body surface area >10%
- Blood urea nitrogen >10 mmol/L (10 mEq/L)
- Serum bicarbonate <20 mmol/L (20 mEq/L)
- Blood glucose >14 mmol/L (252 mg/dL)

    2. Mortality rates based upon the number of positive criteria are as follows:

- 0 to 1 factor = 3%
- 2 factors = 12%
- 3 factors = 35%
- 4 factors = 58%
- 5 or more factors = 90%

Toxic Shock Syndrome

A. *Emergency—call a consult immediately!*

B. Pertinent information: age of patient, immunocompromised status, menstrual history, recent surgeries, diabetes, chronic cardiac or pulmonary disease.

C. Typical signs/symptoms: painful erythematous skin eruption, sudden onset of high fever, nausea/vomiting, diarrhea, sore throat, confusion, headache, myalgias, and hypotension.

D. Physical exam: Fever >102, erythematous rash initially appearing on trunk, spreading to arms and legs, and involving palms and soles, progressing to diffuse erythema and edema, including the oral mucosa. Eventually, there is desquamation of the top layer of the epidermis (not full-thickness as in TEN) in 10–12 days.

E. Work-up: blood cultures, CBC (leukocytosis), blood chemistry profile (hyponatremia, hypokalemia, hypocalcemia, elevated LFTs), ECG (arrhythmias), CXR. To consider: serologic testing for Rocky Mountain spotted fever, leptospirosis, measles, hepatitis B surface antigen, antinuclear antibody, VDRL test, Monospot antibody, rapid strep test, LP (should be normal).

F. Diagnosis: clinical (fever, typical rash, hypotension, multiorgan involvement).

G. Treatment:

   1. Remove any infected foreign bodies.

   2. IV antibiotics effective against streptococcus and penicillinase-resistant *Staphylococcus.* Clindamycin, 900 mg IV q8h for suspected streptococcal TSS; oxacillin 2 g IV q4h for suspected staphylococcal infection (or vancomycin for PCN-allergic patient). Both are usually given until culture confirms the organism.

   3. Aggressive IV fluids.

   4. Consider IVIG.

   5. Monitor for hypotension/shock.

   6. Oxygen therapy

H. Clinical pearls: *Staphylococcus* scalded skin syndrome has a similar clinical picture; however, it occurs in immunocompromised adults. *S. aureus* is the most common cause of TSS; however, exotoxin-producing streptococci can induce a similar clinical picture associated with higher mortality. Clindamycin suppresses synthesis of the TSS toxin (TSST-1) while β-lactamase-resistant antibiotics may increase synthesis of TSST-1. Therefore, the addition of clindamycin (for the first few days of therapy) is recommended with staphylococcal infections.

Necrotizing Fasciitis

A. *Emergency—call a surgeon now!*

B. Pertinent info: recent surgical or traumatic wound.

C. Typical signs and symptoms: Involved area becomes erythematous, indurated, and severely painful. Within hours it can become dusky blue to black, indicating necrosis. Crepitus can develop because of subcutaneous gas formation.

D. Work-up and diagnosis: culture and sensitivity of wound aspirate, plain x-ray for soft tissue gas, and CT/MRI if clinical diagnosis not obvious or to delineate depth of infection.

E. Treatment:

   1. Wide surgical debridement and tissue culture.

   2. IV antibiotics effective against Gram-negative bacilli, streptococci, and anaerobes. Consider agents effective against MRSA if in an endemic area.

F. Clinical pearls: Time is essential—*call for help immediately!* Mortality rate as high as 25%.

Pemphigus Vulgaris (PV) and Bullous Pemphigoid (BP)

A. Urgent consult.

B. Pertinent info: flaccid or tense bullae, percentage body involved, mucosal involvement.

C. Typical signs and symptoms: flaccid bullae and erosions with mucosal involvement (PV) and pruritus with tense bullae in an elderly person (BP).

D. Work-up and diagnosis: skin biopsy with direct immunofluorescence (BP & PV) and serum for indirect immunofluorescence (PV).

E. Treatment:

   1. PV: prednisone, azathioprine, mycophenolate mofetil, gold.

   2. BP: steroids (topical > systemic), tetracycline, nicotinamide.

F. Clinical pearls: PV is associated with a higher mortality than BP. Thus, PV requires aggressive treatment. Most patients do not require hospitalization unless infected or having difficulty maintaining fluid intake. Causes of blistering diseases include infectious, autoimmune, allergic hypersensitivity, metabolic, paraneoplastic, and genetic.

Vasculitis

A. Urgent consult.

B. Pertinent info: drug history, known connective tissue disease, malignancy, or infection.

C. Typical skin findings: palpable purpura (dark reddish-purple lesions that do not blanch and may blister or ulcerate) on the lower extremities or dependent areas. Eruption may be itchy, painful, or asymptomatic.

D. Work-up: CBC, CMP, urinalysis, hemoccult, skin biopsy, CXR, throat culture for strep, ESR, hepatitis panel, cryoglobulins, ANA, RF, antiphospholipid, ANCA, SPEP.

E. Diagnosis: skin biopsy; concern for systemic involvement if fever, arthralgias, abdominal pain, pulmonary symptoms, hematuria, or proteinuria.

F. Treatment:

1. Discontinue potential causative drug (ASA, sulfonamides, penicillin, barbiturates, amphetamines, PTU).
2. Treat underlying disorder (infection, malignancy, or connective tissue disease).
3. Antihistamines, NSAIDs, colchicine, dapsone, antimalarials.
4. Systemic involvement: prednisone, azathioprine, cyclophosphamide, IVIG, plasmapheresis.

G. Clinical pearls: up to 50% of cases are idiopathic. Thrombocytopenia is associated with nonpalpable purpura. DIC and Coumadin necrosis cause extensive purpura. Neisseria sepsis and Rocky Mountain spotted fever also cause petechiae and purpura. Acral hemorrhagic papules, pustules, or vesicles may result from septic emboli.

Hypersensitivity Syndrome (Severe Drug Reaction)

A. Urgent consult.

B. Pertinent information: drug history (sulfonamides, anticonvulsants, allopurinol).

C. Physical exam: blanchable erythematous macules, exfoliative dermatitis, or erythema multiforme (target-like) lesions mostly on the trunk and proximal extremities, fever, lymphadenopathy, hepatosplenomegaly.

D. Work-up: CBC, liver function panel, urinalysis, CXR.

E. Treatment:

1. Stop drug.
2. Oral/topical steroids and antihistamines for symptoms.

F. Clinical pearls: The syndrome develops within 8 weeks of starting the causative drug. Up to 50% develop fulminant hepatic necrosis if the drug is not stopped early in the course. Some anticonvulsants cross react in 70% to 80% of patients (phenytoin, carbamazepine, and phenobarbital). Valproic acid does not cross-react. Patients should warn first-degree relatives that they, too, may be at high risk for a reaction due to an inherited component.

Erythroderma (Generalized Exfoliative Dermatitis)

A. Urgent consult.

B. Pertinent info: prior skin disorder, drug history, duration of erythroderma.

C. Physical exam: diffuse erythema of skin leading to exfoliative dermatitis, pruritus, keratoderma, shivering/chills, alopecia.

D. Most common causes: idiopathic, drug allergy, lymphoma and leukemia (including cutaneous T-cell lymphoma), atopic dermatitis (eczema), psoriasis, contact dermatitis, seborrheic dermatitis.

E. Labs: CBC, blood chemistry panel, albumin, calcium, SPEP, peripheral blood smear for Sézary cells.

F. Diagnosis: clinical, skin biopsy.

G. Treatment:

1. Treat underlying skin condition if known (psoriasis, eczema, etc.).

2. Discontinue suspect drugs if any.

3. Search for and treat underlying malignancy.

4. Topical steroid ointment (midpotency: e.g., triamcinolone 0.1% ointment), emollients, systemic antihistamines.

5. Monitor closely for electrolyte and fluid imbalances, high-output cardiac failure, renal failure, sepsis, and hypothermia.

H. Clinical pearls: 20% of cases are idiopathic. The course and prognosis depend on the underlying etiology. A diligent search for the underlying cause is often required. Most patients do not require hospitalization unless infected or in high-output cardiac failure.

NEUROLOGY

Acute Focal Neurologic Deficit (Stroke)

A. *Level of Urgency—emergent.* If the time of onset is known to be within 3 hours, call immediately, as the patient may be a candidate for thrombolytic therapy.

B. Pertinent Information: There are two broad categories of stroke:

   1. Ischemic (including TIA)—sudden onset focal neurologic deficit attributable to a vascular territory. Transient ischemic attack (TIA) is a focal deficit that completely resolves within 24 hours. Most clear within 5–10 minutes. Ischemic stroke accounts for more than 80% of strokes.

   2. Hemorrhagic—includes intracerebral hemorrhage and subarachnoid hemorrhage.

C. Symptoms and signs: Stroke causes negative neurologic symptoms, such as weakness, loss of sensation, visual loss, and aphasia. Positive symptoms, such as pain, paresthesias, jerking movements, and hallucinations are rare, and suggest seizure. Headache can occur and is more common with hemorrhagic stroke than ischemic.

D. History:

   1. The exact time of onset is essential information, if it can be determined. It is the time the patient was last seen or was known to be normal, not when they were found with the deficits. If the patient awakens with deficits, consider the time he or she went to sleep as the time of onset.

   2. The time course of symptoms (sudden vs. gradual).

   3. Progression of symptoms (stable, worsening, or improving).

   4. Whether there was a fall associated with onset.

   5. Associated symptoms (severe HA, nausea or vomiting may suggest hemorrhagic stroke).

   6. Any known contraindications for thrombolytics (see below).

   7. Past neurologic, medical, and surgical history.

   8. Patient's medications (especially anticoagulants).

E. Physical exam: Vital signs (especially blood pressure, finger stick blood sugar, and oxygen saturation). Any sign of recent head injury. Oral trauma suggesting unwitnessed seizure. Cardio-pulmonary exam to evaluate for arrhythmia, heart failure, and concurrent cardiac ischemia, as well as to monitor for signs of aspiration. Focused neurologic exam.

F. Work-up: Immediate evaluation consists of a STAT noncontrast head CT to evaluate for hemorrhage, stat ECG, CXR, finger-stick glucose, CBC, chemistry panel, and coagulation panel.

G. Treatment of ischemic stroke:

   1. If the time of onset is well established to be within 3 hours, and there are no contraindications for thrombolysis, then IV TPA is the only approved specific treatment for ischemic stroke. Strong contraindications for TPA include blood pressure >185/110; FSBS >400 or <50; seizure at onset; stroke in the last 3 months; history of intracranial hemorrhage; anticoagulant therapy and INR >1.7 or elevated PTT; platelets <100; recent major surgery within 14 days; head injury within 3 months; GI or GU bleeding within 21 days; lumbar puncture within 14 days; arterial puncture at a noncompressible site within 14 days; rapid improvement of symptoms.

2. Blood pressure management: Generally stroke patients are allowed to be hypertensive to improve perfusion to the ischemic penumbra. Consider treatment of blood pressure if the mean arterial pressure exceeds 130 mm Hg. If they have received TPA, there are tighter blood pressure goals to reduce the risk of hemorrhagic conversion. Treatment of the blood pressure is dependent on the risk of end organ damage (i.e., cardiac ischemia, acute renal failure).

3. Airway management: Intubation may be required if the stroke has compromised level of consciousness to the degree that the patient is unable to maintain an adequate airway. Brainstem involvement should prompt aggressive monitoring for early respiratory failure.

4. Reimaging is required if the patient develops worsening of the neurologic examination. Head CT is sufficient to evaluate for likely causes, such as hemorrhage, midline shift, herniation, and hydrocephalus.

5. Stroke patients are at high risk for DVT, and should be started on prophylactic agents (subcutaneous heparin or low molecular weight heparin) as soon as it is considered safe. Generally, ischemic stroke patients can be started on prophylaxis immediately and hemorrhagic stroke patients after 48 hours.

Seizure

A. *Level of urgency—urgent or emergent.* If the patient experiences multiple seizures or has not returned to baseline, an emergent call is indicated. If the patient has returned to baseline after a single convulsion, neurologic evaluation should be obtained on an urgent basis.

B. Description

1. Status epilepticus is defined as multiple seizures without regaining full consciousness between the episodes, or a single seizure that lasts longer than 5 minutes.

   2. Symptoms and signs of focal brain disease: patients may describe an aura prior to the episode, or have postictal focal weakness.

C. Pertinent history:

   1. Has the patient returned to baseline?

   2. Has the patient had seizures before?

   3. What was the seizure like (description of onset, movements, head turning, eye position, loss of continence, oral trauma)?

   4. Are there any known metabolic derangements (hypoglycemia or hyperglycemia can both cause seizures, for example)? Any known drug or toxic exposure?

   5. Any signs of infection?

   6. Any history of head trauma?

D. Physical exam: Evaluate for signs of head injury, oral trauma, or meningismus. Determine level of consciousness and assess for deficits of cranial nerves or motor function.

E. Work-up: Seizures are usually a symptom of an underlying problem; consider a structural lesion (prior stroke, history of head injury), metabolic derangements (check blood sugar, sodium, calcium, phosphorous, renal function), or infection.

F. Treatment: *most importantly, remain calm.*

   1. Single seizure—if the seizure is ongoing, note the time. Check for level of consciousness, ability to follow commands. Look for forced eye deviation or nystagmus. Protect the patient's airway, but do not insert objects into his or her mouth if convulsing. Turn the patient on his or her side, and pad the bed rails. Provide oxygen by face mask, check vital signs, obtain finger stick blood sugar.

   2. Status epilepticus—if the seizure has been continuous for 5 minutes, or if there have been multiple seizures without full return to baseline, status has developed. This should be considered a neurologic "code." Protect the airway, have an intubation kit available, obtain ABG, cardiac monitor, and pulse oximetry (many of these monitors will be difficult to interpret if there are ongoing convulsions). Ensure redundant IV access. Send code labs to include fingerstick blood sugar, CBC, chemistry, Mg, PO_4, urine and serum toxicology, alcohol level, urinalysis, and drug levels for any anticonvulsants the patient should be taking. Give thiamine 100 mg IV followed immediately by 50 mL of 50% dextrose solution. Do not wait for the results of the blood sugar, as hyperglycemia is transient and far less damaging than prolonged hypoglycemia.

   a. Lorazepam (Ativan) 0.1 mg/kg (4–8 mg) at a rate of 1 mg/min) should be administered IV if possible. PR diazepam (0.5 mg/kg to a maximum of 20 mg), or IM midazolam (0.2 mg/kg) can be given if there is no IV access. This should be repeated if there continues to be seizure activity.

   b. An IV anticonvulsant should rapidly follow the benzodiazepine, usually phenytoin (15–20 mg/kg). Blood pressure and cardiac rhythm will need to be monitored. The maximal infusion rate is 50 mg/min. Alternatively, fosphenytoin can be used. It can be infused at rates up to 150 mg/min, and has less risk of hypotension and arrhythmia, but is a pro–drug that must be converted prior to becoming an active anticonvulsant. The cost of fosphenytoin is significantly higher than phenytoin.

3. If the patient continues to have refractory seizures, efforts should be made to transfer them to an ICU with EEG monitoring. Aggressive anticonvulsant therapy requiring intubation and mechanical ventilation may be necessary.

4. Watch for rhabdomyolysis and hyperthermia as complications of prolonged convulsions.

Meningitis

A. *Level of urgency—emergent*

B. Pertinent Information: Bacterial meningitis usually presents with rapidly progressive encephalopathy, headaches, and/or seizures, and is a neurologic emergency. Viral meningitis/encephalitis generally follows a more benign clinical course; however, it also can leave patients with severe neurologic deficits if not recognized and treated early. In HIV and other immunocompromised patients, fungal infections such as cryptococcus also should be considered.

C. History: Patients with bacterial meningitis frequently complain of generalized myalgias, sore throat, and/or fatigue prior to the major clinical deterioration that brings them to medical attention. Fever, headache, and alteration in level of consciousness are common presenting features. Seizures may also be a presenting feature of the infection, as well as photophobia. An acute confusional state in a febrile patient should always raise the consideration for bacterial meningitis. Viral meningitis usually presents with symptoms of altered consciousness, fever, personality changes, headache, and flu-like symptoms. Remember to ask the patient about any recent travel or sick contacts.

D. Physical exam: Evaluation of mental status is essential. Meningeal signs should be checked: Brudzinski's sign (neck flexion resulting in spontaneous flexion of the knees) and Kernig's sign (passive extension of the knees with hips flexed resulting in eye opening and verbal response). Papilledema suggests increased intracranial pressure, which may result from brain edema or sagittal sinus thrombosis. Rash may suggest a specific infectious etiology, typically *Neisseria meningitides*.

E. Work-up: Neuroimaging should be obtained to rule out a mass as the cause of the altered mental status (especially if there is focality on neurologic exam). Blood cultures and urgent lumbar puncture are required. See Table 17-1 for CSF interpretation.

F. Treatment: Antibiotics should not be withheld if the head CT and lumbar puncture are not able to be obtained rapidly. Obtain blood cultures prior to starting antibiotics, as a significant percentage of bacterial meningitis patients will have bacteremia. Antibiotic coverage should include ceftriaxone 2 g q12h, vancomycin 1 g q12h. Ampicillin can be considered for patients at risk for *Listeria*. If viral meningitis is suspected, start acyclovir 10 mg/kg q8h (unless renal impairment) empirically while the HSV PCR is pending. The PCR will remain positive for several days after initiating treatment, so acyclovir should not be delayed. See Table 17-2 for additional treatment recommendations.

Toxidromes

A. *Level of urgency—emergent*

B. Pertinent information:

1. Neuroleptic malignant syndrome (NMS) is suggested when a patient presents with altered mental status, fever, rigidity, and a history of neuroleptic use.

2. Serotonin syndrome appears similar clinically with less rigidity and a history of serotoninergic medication use.

C. Signs and symptoms: Both NMS and serotonin syndrome cause delirium, depressed level of consciousness, tremor, dysautonomia, and fever. Patients with NMS are more likely to have rigidity, and those with serotonin syndrome are more likely to be hyperreflexic with possible clonus. In severe cases of either syndrome seizures may develop.

D. History: Focused on the use of centrally acting medications, and any recent medication dose changes. NMS can be precipitated by the acute withdrawal of antiparkinson medications.

TABLE 17-1 CSF ANALYSIS

Condition	Color	Pressure (mm H_2O)	Cells (No/mL)	Protein (mg/dL)	Glucose (mg/dL)
Normal	Clear	70–180	0–5 mononuclear	15–45	45–80 (two-thirds of serum glucose)
Bacterial meningitis	Opalescent	Increased (may be normal)	>5 to many 1,000 PMNs	50–1,500	0–45
Viral infection	Clear or opalescent	Normal (may be slightly increased)	>5–2,000, mostly lymphs	20–200	Normal (may be slightly decreased)
Tuberculous meningitis	Clear or opalescent	Increased (may be normal	>5–500 lymphs	45–500	10–45
Fungal meningitis	Clear or opalescent	Normal or increased	>5–800 lymphs	Normal or increased	Normal or decreased
Carcinomatous meningitis	Clear or opalescent	Normal or increased	>5–1,000 mononuclear	Up to 500	Normal or decreased
Subarachnoid hemorrhage	Bloody or xanthochromic	Increased (may be normal)	Many RBC; ratio of WBC/RBC same as blood	Up to 2,000	Normal

TABLE 17-2 TREATMENT OPTIONS FOR BACTERIAL MENINGITIS

Age or Clinical Setting	Likely Organism	Empiric Treatment
Immunocompetent 18–50 years	*Streptococcus pneumoniae, Neisseria meningitidis*	Third generation cephalosporin
>50 years	*S. pneumoniae, L. monocytogenes,* Gram-negative bacilli	Third generation cephalosporin + ampicillin
TB	*Mycobacterium tuberculosis*	Isoniazid + rifampin + ethambutol + pyrazinamide
Head trauma, CSF shunt, neurosurgery	Staphylococci, Gram-negative bacilli, *S. pneumoniae*	Vancomycin + ceftazidime
Immunocompromised	*L. monocytogenes,* Gram-negative bacilli; also *S. pneumoniae* and *Haemophilus influenzae*	Ampicillin + ceftazidime
HIV	*Cryptococcus neoforms*	Amphotericin B + flucytosine

E. Physical exam: Patients have clouded sensorium, hyperthermia, and unstable vital signs due to autonomic involvement. They may be hyperreflexic or hypertonic.

F. Work-up: The primary tool in evaluation is the history of medication use (or change in dose). Meningitis, encephalitis, and systemic infection should be excluded.

G. Treatment: For both syndromes management is largely supportive along with prompt withdrawal of the offending medication. Hyperthermia can be corrected with antipyretics, and cooling blankets. Severe hyperthermia results from increased neuromuscular tone and may require treatment with neuromuscular blocking agents. Close observation for signs of autonomic dysfunction is required. Benzodiazepines can be used to reduce agitation. Fluid status and electrolytes should be monitored as either syndrome may cause rhabdomyolysis.

    1. Neuroleptic malignant syndrome may be treated with dopaminergic agents such as bromocriptine or levodopa. Dantrolene may be useful for severe cases.

    2. Serotonin syndrome may respond to cyproheptadine in severe cases.

OBSTETRICS AND GYNECOLOGY

The OB/GYN History and Physical
(please do one before calling a consult)

A. Gynecological history.

    1. Obtain a menstrual history including LMP, pregnancy status, age at menarche, duration between menses, length of menses, amount of vaginal bleeding (i.e., how many pads soaked in how many hours).

    2. History of abnormal Pap smear results?

    3. History of any postmenopausal bleeding?

    4. Obtain a sexual history including number of partners, forms of contraception used currently and in the past, history of any sexually transmitted infections, dyspareunia or bleeding with intercourse.

B. Obstetric history: Gravida and para status, including full-term deliveries, premature deliveries, stillbirths, abortions or miscarriages, and living children (e.g., a patient with two full-term vaginal deliveries and a miscarriage at 8 weeks would be a G3P2012).

C. Physical exam: A thorough exam includes a speculum exam, as well as a bimanual exam, with or without a rectovaginal exam, as indicated. This exam can usually be done at the bedside if access to a pelvic exam table is limited.

　1. Speculum exam: Tools needed: speculum, light source, cotton-tipped applicator, empty red-top test tube, GC/chlamydia probe, microscope, microscope slide, cover slip, normal saline, and potassium hydroxide, if available. pH paper will also help you. Ensure the patient's privacy before you start. You can use a lubricant to make the speculum exam less uncomfortable for your patient. Try to visualize the cervix and note any friability or discharge from the cervical os. Ectocervical secretions can be removed with a large swab and discarded. If you suspect a sexually transmitted disease, place the GC/chlamydia probe gently in the cervical os for approximately 10–20 seconds and remove. Then gently swab the cotton-tipped applicator in the vagina to obtain a sample of the discharge, and store this in the empty red-top tube. Remove the speculum and perform a bimanual exam.

　2. Making a wet prep: Bring your red-top tube to the nearest microscope room and place a small amount of normal saline into the tube to dilute the cells. You can then spread this sample onto a microscope, place a cover slip over it, and view the sample under 10 and 40 power. Comment on any white blood cells, clue cells, red blood cells, and presence of yeast hyphae. You can make a separate slide with a small amount of KOH to perform a whiff test, and then to better visualize the yeast.

Vaginal Discharge

Yeast Vaginitis (Typically Candida albicans)

A. Pertinent information: History typically includes a white, "cheesy" discharge; severe itching; painful intercourse; and a rash or vaginal inflammation. Risk factors include antibiotic use, pregnancy, and diabetes.

B. Diagnosis:

　1. Discharge can vary from watery to homogeneously thick.

　2. pH is usually normal (<4.5).

　3. Budding yeast forms or mycelia appear in up to 80% of cases.

　4. Whiff test is usually negative.

　5. A presumptive diagnosis can be made in the absence of fungal elements, as long as the pH and wet prep results are normal, and the patient has increased erythema or discharge on pelvic/speculum exam. However, if the physical exam is normal and the findings of the wet prep are normal, you should not empirically treat the patient.

C. Treatment:

1. Options include topical medications such as miconazole 2% cream (available in 3- and 7-day preparations), clotrimazole cream, or fluconazole 150 mg PO × one dose.

2. Complicated infections (for patients with recurrent or severe symptoms who are immunocompromised) can be treated with an additional dose of fluconazole given 72 hours within the first dose, or prolonged topical regimens lasting up to 14 days.

3. Diabetic patients may have atypical strains of yeast, such as *C. glabrata.* If there is no response to the initial treatment listed above, refractory infections are often managed with boric acid suppositories (600 mg PV qhs × 2 weeks).

Bacterial Vaginosis (BV)

A. Pertinent information: This is the most common form of vaginitis in the United States, and is frequently caused by *Gardnerella vaginalis* or *Haemophilus vaginalis.* Patients often report a foul-smelling, fish-like odor with a thin, yellow discharge. There may be a rash or painful intercourse, or odor after intercourse. This is not a sexually transmitted disease, and the patient's partner does not need treatment.

B. Diagnosis:

1. Fishy vaginal odor and discharge.

2. Vaginal secretions appear gray and thinly coat the vaginal walls.

3. pH >4.5 (usually 4.7–5.7).

4. Increased number of clue cells (usually greater than 20% of epithelial cells), and absence of white blood cells.

5. Positive "whiff" test (addition of KOH to vaginal secretions results in an amine-like odor).

C. Treatment: Metronidazole 500 mg PO bid × 7 days, or metronidazole gel, 0.75%, one applicator per vagina once nightly × 5 days.

Trichomoniasis

A. Pertinent Information: Caused by a sexually-transmitted protozoan parasite, *Trichomonas vaginalis.*

B. Diagnosis:

    1. Profuse, purulent malodorous discharge accompanied by vaginal pruritus. Sores can develop on the cervix, and there may be pain on urination or intercourse.

    2. Colpitis macularis ("strawberry cervix") can be observed.

    3. pH usually higher than 5.0.

    4. Saline wet prep reveals motile trichomonads and increased number of white blood cells.

    5. Clue cells may be present, as BV is commonly associated, and the "whiff" test may be positive.

C. Treatment: Metronidazole, either 2 g PO × one dose only, or 500 mg PO bid × 7 days. Metronidazole gel has *not* been shown to be as effective for treatment of trichomoniasis. The patient's sexual partner should be treated as well.

Cervicitis

A. Pertinent information: Most commonly caused by *Neisseria gonorrhea* or *Chlamydia trachomatis*.

B. Diagnosis: Purulent endocervical discharge, generally yellow or green in color. A GC/chlamydia probe can be sent, preferably from the cervical os as described above. If this is not available, a urine probe for GC/chlamydia can also be performed. If you suspect that a patient may have pelvic inflammatory disease due to the presence of cervical motion tenderness, fever, leukocytosis or worsening pelvic pain, an OB/GYN consult should be obtained.

C. Treatment:

    1. *N. gonorrhea*:

        a. Ceftriaxone 125 mg IM × one dose (preferred).

        b. Cefiximine 400 mg PO × one dose.

        c. Fluoroquinalones are no longer recommended due to high resistance rates.

        d. Always treat for *C. trachomatis* if not already ruled out!

    2. *C. trachomatis:*

        a. Azithromycin 1 g PO × one dose.

        b. Doxycycline 100 mg PO bid × 7 days.

Ectopic Pregnancy

A. *A ruptured ectopic pregnancy is a true obstetric emergency and your consulting OB/GYN team should be notified immediately.*

B. History: Date of patient's LMP and menstrual history, type of contraception (if any), history of tubal ligation (*Note: History of a tubal ligation does not by any means rule out an ectopic pregnancy; in fact it increases the chance of an ectopic, if the patient becomes pregnant again*), history of previous ectopic pregnancy, amount of vaginal bleeding (if any), and degree of abdominal pain (if any).

C. Physical exam/work-up:

1. Take **vital signs immediately** with orthostatics. Depending on the gestational age, fetal heart tones may be auscultated by Doppler, but a pelvic ultrasound, performed both transabdominally and transvaginally, is key to making this diagnosis.

2. Tests to be drawn include CBC, type and cross, and a urine pregnancy test. If the urine pregnancy test is positive, draw a serum quantitative β-hCG immediately.

D. Treatment:

1. Place large-bore IV immediately. If the patient is hypotensive, resuscitate with IV fluids and blood products as necessary.

2. Treatment for ectopic pregnancy can be medical (with methotrexate) or surgical (with laparoscopic or open salpingectomy or salpingostomy), depending on the patient's stability and characteristics of the ectopic. Before any treatment decisions are made, consultation should be made with the OB/GYN team.

Vaginal Bleeding

A. Pertinent information: The differential diagnosis of vaginal bleeding includes the following:

1. Exogenous hormones.

2. Endocrine imbalances (hyper- or hypothyroidism, diabetes).

3. Anatomic (fibroids, polyps, cervical lesions).

4. Coagulopathies and other hematologic causes.

5. Infectious causes (cervicitis).

6. Neoplasia.

7. Dysfunctional uterine bleeding (a diagnosis of exclusion, when no specific cause can be found) (Table 17-3).

B. History: It is important to assess how long the bleeding has lasted, where the patient is in her cycle, how much bleeding has occurred, if there is a history of bleeding disorders, and whether the patient is on hormones, contraception, or anticoagulants. Also note when she last took any of these medications, or if any of the medication has been recently changed.

TABLE 17-3 CAUSES OF BLEEDING BY APPROXIMATE FREQUENCY AND AGE GROUP

Adolescent	Reproductive	Perimenopausal	Postmenopausal
Anovulation	Exogenous hormone use	Anovulation	Exogenous hormone use
Exogenous hormone use	Pregnancy	Fibroids	Endometrial lesions, including cancer
			Atrophic vaginitis
Pregnancy	Anovulation	Cervical and endometrial polyps	Other tumor
Coagulopathy	Fibroids	Thyroid dysfunction	
	Cervical and endometrial polyps		
	Thyroid dysfunction		

Adapted from Berek JS. *Berek and Novak's Gynecology.* 14th ed. Philadelphia: Lippincott, Williams and Wilkins, 2007.

C. Physical exam: A gynecologic exam, including a speculum exam and pelvic exam, should be performed in order to determine the extent and source of bleeding. Make sure the bleeding is from the vagina or uterus and not the urethra (inspect the urethra), bladder (do a straight catheterization with a urinalysis), or rectum (rectal exam).

D. Work-up: Appropriate laboratory studies include a CBC to detect anemia or thrombocytopenia and a pregnancy test in reproductive-aged women. In certain individuals a TSH and screening coagulation studies may be appropriate to rule out thyroid dysfunction or a primary coagulation problem, respectively. Consider testing for von Willebrand's disease, especially in adolescent women (bleeding time or platelet function analyzer [PFA] testing). Women with chronic anovulation, obesity, or age greater than 35 require further evaluation. A vaginal ultrasound can be helpful in assessing for anatomic abnormalities, and assessment of the endometrial stripe thickness is useful in postmenopausal women. Endometrial sampling, accomplished in the office using disposable plastic cannulae, should be performed in these women, as they are at risk for polyps, hyperplasia, or carcinoma of the endometrium.

E. Treatment:

1. **Heavy** vaginal bleeding can be an emergency; this should be assessed immediately, and you should have a low threshold to call a consult. First, though, type and cross the patient for at least 2 units of PRBCs and make sure a pregnancy test has been done and a large-bore IV has been placed.

2. Correct any underlying coagulation disorder and discontinue anticoagulants, if possible.

3. If anovulatory bleeding is established as the working diagnosis, hormonal therapy with PO (2.5 mg q6h) or IV estrogen (25–40 mg q6h) will usually control bleeding, but start this in consultation with the OB/GYN team. If hormonal management fails, a local cause of bleeding is more likely.

4. In most cases, abnormal bleeding can be managed medically. Hormonal management, including low-dose oral contraceptives, can be used to significantly reduce blood flow. When estrogen is contraindicated, progestins can be used, including cyclic oral medroxyprogesterone acetate, depot forms of medroxyprogesterone acetate, and the levonorgestrel-containing intrauterine device, which has been shown to decrease menstrual blood loss by 80% to 90%.

5. Surgical management ranges from endometrial ablation, hysteroscopy with resection of uterine polyps or leiomyomas, myomectomy, uterine artery embolization, magnetic resonance-guided focused ultrasonography ablation, and, most definitively, hysterectomy.

Pelvic Mass

A. *Call a gynecology consult immediately for suspected ovarian torsion.* Other causes do not require emergent consultation.

B. History: Obtain a thorough history including menstrual history, menopausal status, pregnancy status, history of neoplasia, history of vaginal bleeding, last Pap smear, history or recent biopsy of any gynecologic organs, and history of any gynecologic surgery. Ask about family history of ovarian, breast, or colon cancer, and history of tobacco use.

C. Differential diagnosis: A variety of entities may result in the formation of a pelvic mass. These may be gynecologic in origin, or may arise from the urinary tract or bowel. Gynecologic causes of a pelvic mass may be uterine, adnexal, or more specifically ovarian. Table 17-4 outlines the most common causes of pelvic masses for each age group. Age is an important determinant of the likelihood of malignancy.

D. Physical exam: A complete pelvic exam, including a rectovaginal exam and Pap test, should be performed. Evidence of ascites or a pleural effusion heightens the suspicion for a malignant ovarian tumor.

E. Work-up: Pelvic ultrasonography, usually done transvaginally, will help to clarify the origin of the mass, whether it is uterine, adnexal, urinary, or gastrointestinal. Endometrial sampling with an endometrial biopsy or dilatation and curettage is necessary if both a pelvic mass and abnormal bleeding are present. Laboratory studies should include cervical cytology, complete blood count, testing of stool for occult blood, and a pregnancy test in reproductive-age women. CA-125 is a nonspecific tumor marker that may be obtained, but be aware that a number of benign conditions, including leiomyomas, PID, pregnancy, and endometriosis can cause elevated levels of this marker. A barium enema or other study of the GI tract will help to exclude a gastrointestinal etiology.

F. Clinical pearl: Ovarian torsion may present as a pelvic mass but is usually accompanied by intermittent severe abdominal pain,

TABLE 17-4 MOST COMMON CAUSES OF PELVIC MASSES FOR EACH AGE GROUP

Adolescent	Reproductive	Perimenopausal	Postmenopausal
Functional cyst	Functional cyst	Fibroids	Ovarian tumor (malignant or benign)
Pregnancy	Pregnancy	Epithelial ovarian tumor	Functional cyst
Dermoid/other germ cell tumors	Uterine fibroids	Functional cyst	Bowel, malignant tumor or inflammatory
Obstructing vaginal or uterine anomalies	Epithelial ovarian tumor		Metastases
Epithelial ovarian tumor			

Adapted from Berek JS. Berek and Novak's Gynecology. 14th ed. Philadelphia: Lippincott, Williams and Wilkins, 2007.

tender pelvic mass by exam, and low-grade temperatures, and on pelvic ultrasound may be accompanied by decreased flow to the ovary. Ovarian torsion is a surgical emergency, and promptly consulting the OB/GYN service can mean the difference between a young woman losing her ovary versus being able to preserve it. Presence of a pelvic mass makes torsion more likely, but keep in mind that a normal ovary can torse as well.

OPHTHALMOLOGY

Trauma with Possible Ruptured Globe

A. *Ocular emergency—call a consult immediately!*

B. Pertinent information: age, PMH/PSH/ocular history, allergies, current meds including ocular meds, specific ocular complaints, history of events preceding trauma, specific chemicals or items involved, any history of possible foreign body (e.g., hammering on metal).

C. Typical symptoms: pain, decreased vision, history of trauma.

D. Physical exam findings: 360 degree subconjunctival hemorrhage, full-thickness corneal or scleral laceration, peaked or irregular pupil, exposed intraocular contents, hyphema (bleeding in the anterior chamber).

E. Treatment:
   1. Place a shield over the involved eye; **do not press on eye or touch ocular contents.**
   2. NPO (determine last meal).
   3. IV antibiotics: cefazolin or vancomycin 1 g IV immediately; also give fluoroquinolone—ciprofloxacin, gatifloxacin, or moxifloxacin 400 mg PO or IV.
   4. Administer tetanus toxoid as needed.
   5. Antiemetic as needed to prevent Valsalva.
   6. Orbital CT scan (axial and coronal).
   7. Surgical repair as soon as possible.

E. Clinical pearls:
   1. In trauma with eyelid laceration; *do not* try to repair the laceration. Allow ophthalmologist to assess extent.
   2. Significant orbital trauma may require evaluation for retrobulbar hemorrhage, optic nerve trauma, and fractures.

Injury

Acute Chemical Splash

A. *Ocular emergency*—begin irrigation, *then call a consult immediately.*

B. Pertinent information: age, PMH/PSH/ocular history, allergies, current meds including ocular meds, specific ocular complaints, history of events, specific chemicals or items involved, time/duration of contact, whether irrigated at the scene.

C. Symptoms: ± pain, blurry vision, foreign body sensation, tearing, photophobia.

D. Physical exam:

1. Mild to moderate splash: Sloughing of entire epithelium, hyperemia, mild chemosis (edema of bulbar conjunctiva), eyelid edema, first- or second-degree periocular skin burns.

2. Moderate to severe: Pronounced chemosis, perilimbal (at the junction of cornea and sclera) blanching, corneal edema or opacification, anterior chamber reaction/no view of the anterior chamber, increased intraocular pressure, second- or third-degree burns.

E. Work-up: Slit-lamp exam, evert eyelids, check pH, intraocular pressure.

F. Immediate treatment:

1. *Copious irrigation* with 1 L of any available irrigant (e.g., NS, 1/2 NS, or LR), and *keep irrigating* until you talk with the consultant.

2. May give 1–2 drops of topical anesthetic.

3. Do *not* use acid or alkali to neutralize splash.

4. Check pH 5 minutes after irrigation; continue irrigation until pH is neutral (i.e., 7).

G. Treatment *after* irrigation (ideally instituted by ophthalmologist):

1. Debride necrotic tissue.

2. Topical antibiotic ointment: bacitracin/polymyxin (Polysporin), erythromycin, or ciprofloxacin (Ciloxan) ophthalmic qid.

3. Cycloplege (temporarily paralyzes the ciliary muscles) the eye with scopolamine 0.25% tid (avoid phenylephrine).

4. Topical steroid: prednisolone 1% (Pred Forte) qid (do not start steroids unless patient followed by ophthalmology).

5. Acetazolamide 250 mg PO qid if intraocular pressure is increased.

6. Frequent (~q1h) preservative-free artificial tears.

7. Daily follow-up with ophthalmology; gradual taper of steroids.

Corneal Ulcer
A. *This is an emergency—call a consult immediately.*
B. Pertinent information: age, past ocular history, history leading up to event (recent trauma or contact lens use).
C. Symptoms: pain, photophobia, decreased vision, $\pm$ discharge.
D. Physical exam: focal corneal opacity and overlying epithelial defect (abrasion), anterior chamber reaction, $+/-$ hypopyon (white blood cells layering out in anterior chamber), eyelid edema.
E. Work-up: Routine cultures taken of corneal scrapings (done by ophthalmologist)—includes Gram stain, KOH prep, fungal culture.
F. Treatment:
   1. Moxifloxacin (Vigamox) or gatifloxacin (Zymar) drops, q1–4h, and cycloplege with scopolamine 0.25% tid.
   2. If ulcer is severe, patient will be admitted and given topical fortified cefazolin (Ancef) or vancomycin 50 mg/mL 1 drop q hour and tobramycin 15 mg/mL 1 drop q hour.
   3. Daily ophthalmology follow-up.
G. Clinical pearls: Contact lens wearers are at much higher risk. Bacteria, fungi, HSV, and *Acanthamoeba* are all possible causes.

Corneal Abrasion or Foreign Body
A. This is usually not an emergency, but consult if in doubt.
B. Pertinent information: age, past ocular history, history of events leading up to event, occupational history (i.e., grinding, drilling, trauma), contact lens use, type of foreign body.
C. Symptoms: acute pain, tearing, photophobia, foreign body sensation.
D. Work-up:
   1. Blue light or slit-lamp exam with fluorescein to detect epithelial defect (seen as green fluorescent spot).
   2. Look for foreign body or rust ring.
   3. Measure and record dimension of defect.
   4. Evert eyelids to look for hidden foreign bodies.
   5. Look for associated corneal ulcers (white opacity seen before fluorescein instilled).
E. Treatment:
   1. Remove foreign body (preferably by an ophthalmologist).
   2. Noncontact lens wearers: treat with bacitracin/polymyxin (Polysporin) or erythromycin ointment q 2–4h or polymyxin B/trimethoprim (Polytrim) drops tid.

3. Contact lens wearers: Moxifloxacin (Vigamox) or gatifloxacin (Zymar) drops qid or tobramycin or ciprofloxacin ointment q2–4h. No contact lens use until cleared by an ophthalmologist.

4. Cycloplege with cyclopentolate 1% tid if any significant photophobia.

5. Follow up with an ophthalmologist the next day and as needed thereafter.

E. Clinical pearls: If there is any chance of penetrating injury, call a consult immediately.

Acute Vision Loss
Central Retinal Artery Occlusion

A. *Ocular emergency—call a consult STAT! (Like a CVA, "time is vision"!)*

B. Pertinent information: age, PMH/PSH/ocular history, allergies, current meds including ocular meds, specific ocular complaints, history of preceding event, vision loss.

C. Symptoms: painless, unilateral, acute loss of vision, prior history of amaurosis fugax (painless, temporary, uniocular vision loss).

D. Physical exam: whitening of the retina with a "cherry red" spot in the center of the macula, afferent pupillary defect (Marcus Gunn pupil), narrowed arterioles, occasionally arteriolar emboli/plaque visible.

E. Work-up: ESR in patients over 50 years of age, fasting blood sugar, CBC, PT/PTT; in younger patients, also check ANA, RF, FTA-ABS, SPEP, Sickledex, and antiphospholipid antibodies. Check blood pressure. Patient may need carotid Dopplers and cardiac echo.

F. Treatment:

1. Call ophthalmologist! Permanent visual loss likely after 90–120 minutes.

2. Ocular massage: have patient close eyes; apply pressure to the globe for 5–15 seconds, then release. Repeat several times.

G. Clinical pearls:

1. **Ask about symptoms of giant cell arteritis and check ESR in all patients over 50 years of age!**

2. Etiologies include embolus (carotid or cardiac), thrombosis, giant cell arteritis, collagen vascular disease, hypercoagulation disorders, and rare causes (i.e., migraine, Behçet disease, syphilis).

Acute Angle-Closure Glaucoma

A. *Ocular emergency—call a consult immediately!*

B. Pertinent information: age, PMH/PSH/ocular history, allergies, current meds including ocular meds, specific ocular complaints, family history, recent surgery, recent laser surgery.

C. Symptoms: Pain, blurry vision, colored halos around lights, frontal headache, nausea/vomiting.

D. Physical exam: Conjunctival injection; fixed, mid-dilated pupil (usually in one eye); shallow anterior chamber; acutely elevated intraocular pressure (40s or above).

E. Work-up: Slit-lamp exam, measure intraocular pressure.

F. Treatment:

1. Topical antiglaucoma drops (timolol [Timoptic]—avoid if patient has COPD or asthma; brimonidine [Alphagan], dorzolamide [Trusopt], latanoprost [Xalatan]).

2. Topical steroid prednisolone (Pred Forte) 1% q 15min × 4 doses.

3. Carbonic anhydrase inhibitor IV or PO (i.e., acetazolamide [Diamox] 250 mg IV).

4. If patient is phakic (no prior lens removal), give pilocarpine 1%–2%; if aphakic (history of lens removal), use cycloplegic agent such as cyclopentolate 1%–2%. Consult ophthalmology first.

5. Definitive (laser) treatment by ophthalmologist.

G. Clinical pearls: Be aware of patient's cardiovascular and pulmonary status; evaluate electrolyte/renal status before starting carbonic anhydrase inhibitors or osmotic agents. Etiology can be from an anatomic pupillary block, neovascular, anterior displacement of lens–iris diaphragm (i.e., choroidal effusion, tumor), malignant glaucoma, or medications (i.e., mydriatics, anticholinergics).

Papilledema (Disc Edema Secondary to Increased Intracranial Pressure)

A. *Emergency—call a consult immediately!*

B. Pertinent information: age, PMH/PSH/ocular history, allergies, current meds including ocular meds, specific ocular complaints, history of events preceding trauma.

C. Symptoms: transient vision loss ("gray-outs"), headache, nausea/vomiting, diplopia, visual field defects.

D. Physical exam: bilateral swollen, hyperemic discs; blurring of disc margins; obscuration of vessels; normal pupillary response and color vision (can have sixth nerve palsy from increased ICP).

E. Work-up: Check BP; careful ocular exam (pupils, color vision, exam of fundus); urgent orbital and head CT. Consider LP (after head CT), CBC, TSH, ESR. Consider a neurology consult.

F. Treatment: Treat underlying cause!

G. Clinical pearls: Etiologies you may see on a medical service include pseudotumor cerebri, subdural/subarachnoid hemorrhage, AVM or sagittal sinus thrombosis, intracranial tumors, brain abscess, meningitis/encephalitis, hydrocephalus, malignant HTN, uveitis, infiltrative disease (i.e., sarcoid, TB, syphilis), ischemic optic neuropathy (i.e., giant cell arteritis), central retinal vein occlusion, papillitis (i.e., multiple sclerosis/optic neuritis, diabetic eye disease). It is often helpful to communicate the level of confidence of your fundus exam to the consultant.

Retinal Detachment

A. *Ocular urgency—call a consult.*

B. Pertinent information: Age, PMH/PSH/ocular history, allergies, current meds, specific complaints, history of preceding trauma or surgery.

C. Symptoms: Painless unilateral decreased vision with associated flashes and floaters, curtain or veil across vision, relative visual field defect.

D. Physical exam: Typically a "white & quiet" appearing eye—externally looks normal, usually *no* afferent pupillary defect unless a large retinal detachment. Fundus exam reveals a white, billowing, or wrinkled retina.

E. Work-up: Slit-lamp exam and dilated fundus exam.

F. Treatment:

1. No acute intervention.

2. Low level activity.

3. Needs a retina specialist evaluation.

G. Clinical pearls: Risk factors include recent eye surgery, ocular trauma, high myopia, and a retinal detachment in contralateral eye. A peripheral retinal tear or hole may present with only flashes or floaters and no change in vision. These still require urgent ophthalmologic intervention.

Infection

Endophthalmitis (Infection of the Inside of the Eye)

A. *Ocular emergency—call a consult immediately!*

B. Pertinent information: Age, PMH/PSH/ocular history, allergies, current meds including ocular meds, history of ocular surgery or trauma.

C. Symptoms: Unilateral painful eye, decreased vision.

D. Physical exam: Moderate injection, hypopyon (pus behind the cornea), poor red reflex or view to the back of the eye.

E. Treatment:

1. Emergent ophthalmologic evaluation.

2. Admission.

3. May need culture and injected antibiotics.

F. Clinical pearls: A diagnosis of endophthalmitis must be considered *first* in any patient with recent ocular surgery!

Herpes Zoster Virus

A. This is not an ocular emergency, but urgent referral to ophthalmologist is strongly recommended.

B. Pertinent information: Age, PMH, ocular history, immunocompromised/AIDS?

C. History: Skin rash and discomfort, blurred vision, eye pain, red eye?

D. Physical exam: Skin vesicles in dermatomal distribution respecting the midline (Hutchinson sign = if rash involves the tip of the nose, high chance of eye being involved), conjunctivitis, uveitis, scleritis, cranial nerve palsy.

E. Treatment:

1. If younger than 40 years old, evaluate for immunosuppression.

2. Oral antiviral (e.g., acyclovir 800 mg PO 5 times a day) for 7–10 days.

3. Erythromycin ointment to skin lesions bid.

4. Artificial tears or erythromycin ophthalmic ointment to eye as needed.

5. Follow up with ophthalmologist.

The Red Eye (Fig. 17-2)

Conjunctivitis

A. This is not an emergency.

B. Pertinent information: Age, possible contacts, past ocular history, allergies or previous history of allergic conjunctivitis; make sure there is no pain involved for allergic and viral conjunctivitis.

C. Symptoms:

Viral: Unilateral red eye, possible associated URI symptoms, mild itching, morning crusting or discharge.

Allergic: Bilateral itching, mild redness, watery discharge.

Bacterial: Acute purulent discharge, eyelid edema, decreased vision.

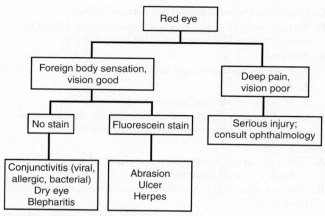

Figure 17-2 Algorithm for red eye.

D. Physical exam:

Viral: Conjunctival injection, crusting, follicles.
Allergic: Lid swelling, chemosis, papillae.
Bacterial: Purulent discharge.

E. Work-up:

Bacterial: Gram stain and culture for *Staphylococcus, Streptococcus, H. flu, N. gonorrhea.*

F. Treatment:

Viral:

1. No specific medical treatment necessary—self-limited illness.
2. Symptomatic treatment with cool compresses or artificial tears.
3. Naphazoline (Naphcon A or Vasocon) may be prescribed tid × 7 days.
4. Wash hands, towels, pillowcases. Use separate towels. No contact lens use until asymptomatic for at least 7 days.
5. Avoid close contact (especially rubbing eyes and touching others) without washing hands first.

Allergic:

1. Eliminate inciting agent.
2. Cool compresses and artificial tears.

3. Olopatadine (Patanol) or nedocromil (Alocril) antihistamine drops bid.

Bacterial:

1. Topical trimethoprim/polymyxin B (Polytrim) or bacitracin ointment qid for 5–7 days.

2. For *H. flu*: Amoxicillin/clavulanate (Augmentin) (20 to 40 mg/kg/day in three divided doses).

3. For GC: Ceftriaxone 1 g IM and empiric treatment for chlamydia with azithromycin 1 g PO × one. Treat sexual partners.

G. Clinical pearls: If vision is acutely and significantly reduced, a diagnosis of conjunctivitis is UNLIKELY. Any pupillary inequality in a patient with red eye(s) is a danger signal for serious ocular disease. Immediate ophthalmologic consultation is warranted in these situations.

Acute Hordeolum (Stye)

A. Not an emergency.

B. Symptoms: Pain, redness, "bump" on lid.

C. Physical exam: Red, tender, swollen nodule around the lid margin or hair follicle.

D. Treatment:

1. Hot compress to eyelids for 5–10 minutes qid.

2. Topical antibiotic such as bacitracin/polymyxin (Polysporin) or erythromycin ophthalmic ointment bid.

3. Follow up with ophthalmologist in 1 week if not resolved.

ORTHOPEDIC SURGERY

General Principles

A. Examination: A thorough examination of the patient should be made *prior* to calling an orthopaedic consult. This should include: neurovascular exam (pulses, sensation, motor function) of involved extremity. *All wounds should also be examined, especially open fractures, diabetic foot ulcerations, and surgical incisions.*

B. Radiography: *Prior* to calling a consult, obtain and evaluate x-rays of the affected joint/bone. Consultation with the orthopedics service is preferred, prior to obtaining a CT or MRI.

C. For all open fractures, suspected compartment syndrome, joint sepsis, cauda equina syndrome, or diabetic infections; *make patients NPO.*

Fractures

A. *Open fractures and fractures with associated neurovascular compromise are emergencies—order x-rays and labs, make patient NPO, and call a consult immediately!*

B. History: Mechanism of injury and pre-injury level of activity.

C. Physical exam: Complete distal neurologic and vascular exam. Examine all wounds: probe w/ Q-tip to determine depth, bone exposure, possible contamination. Examine joints proximal and distal to the fracture. Examine all extremities to rule out other injuries. Take down splints/dressings to perform exams.

D. Work-up: Usually AP and lateral views are sufficient. The following list contains some common fractures in which additional views are necessary for diagnosis, preop planning, or both. Remember to always order plain films prior to a CT or MRI.

   1. Shoulder/proximal humerus: AP, true AP, axillary, scapular lateral (or Y) views.

   2. Hip Fractures (Femoral neck/intertrochanteric fractures): AP hip, cross-table lateral, AP ortho pelvis, AP and lateral femur.

   3. Pelvis/Acetabular fractures: AP ortho pelvis, Judet (oblique) views, inlet/outlet views.

   4. Ankle: AP, lateral, mortise.

   5. Foot: AP, lateral, medial oblique; Harris heel (axial) view if a calcaneal fracture is suspected.

E. Describing fractures: Attempt to delineate the following *prior* to calling consultation.

   1. Fracture pattern (transverse, oblique, spiral).

   2. Displacement. (How far are the fragments away from each other? Which direction: anterior, posterior, medial, lateral?)

   3. Angulation (by how many degrees the fragments relate to each other).

   4. Shortening (how much the fragments overlap).

   5. Comminution (Is it a "clean" break, or are there multiple small fragments about the fracture site?).

   6. Open versus closed: Using a Q-tip, determine the size of the wound, depth, presence of exposed bone/fracture, and neurovascular status (sensation, pulses, motor intact?).

F. Initial treatment/management:

   1. Open fractures require emergent operative debridement and fixation.

2. Keep patients NPO.
3. Establish tetanus status. Give tetanus booster, as needed.
4. Give IV antibiotics (*if fracture is open*) according to fracture grade:
   a. Grade I fractures (1 cm wound and smaller): cefazolin.
   b. Grade II fractures (>1 to 10 cm): cefazolin and gentamicin.
   c. Grade III fracture (>10 cm): cefazolin, gentamicin, and Flagyl.
5. Closed fractures are treated on an individual basis based on particular bone involvement and amount of displacement.
6. DVT prophylaxis: For all patients, place TEDs/SCDs to lower extremities (except if injured). Discuss w/ orthopaedic consult before beginning heparin, subcutaneous low molecular weight heparin, etc.

Septic Joint

A. *This is an **emergency**—call an orthopaedic consult immediately after complete examination, x-rays, and labs obtained. MAKE PATIENT NPO.*

B. Pertinent history: Warmth, painful range-of-motion, tenderness, fever. Inability to ambulate/use extremity.

C. Pertinent exam: Neurovascular exam (pulses, sensation, motor), effusion/fluctuance, erythema, warmth. *Considerable* pain with range-of-motion.

D. Work-up: Plain radiographs, CBC, BMP, ESR, CRP, and blood cultures (if febrile). The diagnosis is confirmed with joint aspiration. Aspiration may be done by the primary physician or an orthopedics consultant. Synovial fluid should be sent for stat Gram stain, cell count, crystals, and cultures (aerobic and anaerobic).

Antibiotics should not be administered until a joint aspirate is obtained.

F. Diagnosis:

1. Septic arthritis is diagnosed with a synovial fluid leukocyte count generally >50,000 per cubic mm, a positive Gram stain, or a positive culture result.
2. An inflammatory/autoimmune arthropathy typically has a synovial fluid leukocyte count of 10,000–50,000 per cubic mm with positive crystals (for gout or CPPD disease), and negative Gram's stain and culture results.

F. Treatment:

1. Operative drainage. (*Neisseria* species [*gonorrhoeae* and *meningitides*] are exceptions to this rule, as they are highly responsive to antibiotic therapy; operative debridement is not necessary.)

2. Appropriate intravenous antibiotics as determined by cultures. The course of antibiotics is typically 6 weeks total. Consider an infectious diseases consult and long term venous access (e.g., PICC line or tunneled central venous catheter) if intravenous antibiotics are needed.

3. Make the patient NPO upon *suspicion* of septic arthritis. Only allow patient to take PO *after* infection has been ruled out. Begin perioperative management and obtain pre-operative labs as indicated (e.g., CBC, BMP, coags, type and screen).

G. Clinical pearls: *S. aureus* is the most common organism in septic arthritis. *N. gonorrhoeae* is also prevalent in sexually active adolescents and adults, whereas *Salmonella* is more common in patients with sickle cell disease.

Compartment Syndrome

A. *Compartment syndrome is an* **emergency**—*call a consult immediately after complete examination and x-rays.*

B. Definition: Compartment syndromes are caused by elevated hydrostatic pressure within a fascial compartment, leading to tissue ischemia as compartment pressure exceeds capillary pressure (i.e., the pressure in the compartment prevents blood flow out of and into the affected area). Elevated hydrostatic pressure commonly occurs from bleeding or swelling from within the compartment.

C. When to consider this: The most specific signs and symptoms of compartment syndrome are pain out of proportion to injury, pain with passive stretch of the muscles in the involved compartment, and hard tense compartments. Paraesthesias, pallor, pulselessness, and paralysis may or may not be present. *All external circumferential dressings should be removed before examining a patient for compartment syndrome.*

D. History: A typical history may include the following:

1. Trauma (fracture or muscle contusion).
2. Ischemia (vascular injury, extended compression).
3. Venous obstruction.
4. Massive inflammation from snake or insect bites.
5. Bleeding into the compartment (consider in anticoagulated patients).

6. Infiltration of fluid into a compartment (paint gun injuries, IV infiltration).

7. Tight circumferential dressings.

E. Physical exam: Directly palpate the concerning area to determine "tightness" of compartments. Passively range the muscles that traverse the compartment (i.e., in the forearm, passively flex and extend the fingers). Check for pulses, sensation, and motor function. Continue to monitor the patient with serial exams.

F. When clinical signs are equivocal, compartment pressures may be measured by an orthopedics consultant. Compartment pressures >30 mm Hg (or a diastolic blood pressure to compartment pressure difference <30 mm Hg in hypotensive patients) are diagnostic for compartment syndrome.

G. Treatment: Make patient NPO immediately upon *suspicion of diagnosis*. Obtain plain x-rays and any indicated pre-op labs (CBC, BMP, coags, T&C 2 units PRBC). Begin perioperative management for emergent fasciotomy by orthopedics team.

H. Clinical pearls: Remember that rhabdomyolysis can occur with compartment syndrome from muscle necrosis. Follow urine output, creatinine, and CPK.

Acute Cauda Equina Syndrome

A. *This is an* **emergency**—*call a consult immediately after examination and x-rays.*

B. Definition: Cauda equina syndrome is an injury to the spinal canal located between the conus and the lumbosacral nerve roots, resulting in bowel and bladder dysfunction, saddle anesthesia, severe lower extremity neurologic deficit, and anal sphincter laxity.

C. History: Suspect in a patient with low back pain and the previously mentioned signs and symptoms.

D. Physical exam: A complete lower extremity neurologic exam should be performed including lower extremity strength, sensation, and reflexes. A rectal exam should also be performed to assess both rectal tone and perianal sensation. Remember that the cauda equina functions as the peripheral nervous system. Therefore, in a complete cauda equina injury, all peripheral nerves to the bowel, bladder, perianal area, and lower extremities will be lost, resulting in absent bulbocavernosus, anal wink, and lower extremity reflexes.

E. Work-up: STAT AP and lateral views of the lumbar spine and a STAT MRI of the lumbar spine. If the patient has had a prior discectomy, obtain MRI with gadolinium contrast. If the patient has had previous spinal surgery with instrumentation, obtain a CT myelogram.

F. Treatment: Keep patient NPO, obtain necessary preoperative blood work, and discontinue anticoagulants. Begin perioperative management for emergent operative decompression.

Diabetic Foot Ulcer/Infections

A. Pertinent information: The acuity of these infections is dictated by the patient's systemic symptoms. *If the patient is febrile and/or unstable, call a consult immediately.*

B. Definition: Diabetic ulcerations occur after patients lose the protective sensation in their feet. Patients may present with an advanced infection due to lack of pain. Neuropathic ulcers typically develop on the plantar surfaces of the feet.

C. History: Recent glycemic control (fingerstick blood glucoses), prior amputations or debridements, history of renal dysfunction.

D. Physical examination: Obtain a thorough neurovascular exam including pulses, sensation, and motor function. Examine all wounds taking note of depth, purulence, necrotic tissue, exposed bone, and proximal extension. If peripheral pulses are absent or diminished, perform and ankle arm index (AAI) and *consider vascular surgery consult* (see "Ischemic Ulcer of the Lower Extremity" in the General Surgery section).

E. Work-up: CBC, BMP, coagulation panel, ESR, and CRP. Obtain AP, lateral, and oblique views of the ankle and foot. *Do not obtain an MRI prior to an orthopedics consult.*

F. Treatment: Surgical management will vary based on the wound and can range from bedside debridement to limb amputation. Antimicrobial therapy should be based upon tissue or bone culture results when possible, but broad spectrum agents (e.g., pipercillin/tazobactam or meropenem +/− vancomycin) should be started promptly for signs of hemodynamic compromise. Consider an infectious diseases consultation, as well as placement of a long-term venous access device if an extended course of intravenous antibiotics is anticipated.

OTOLARYNGOLOGY

Airway Emergencies

A. *Call a consult or the airway pager immediately for assistance!*

B. Pertinent history: Note onset, duration, progression, and severity of stridor (the degree of stridor may not necessarily indicate the severity of obstruction). Does it occur with inspiration, expiration, or both? Are there voice changes? History of prior intubation, neck trauma, head and neck surgery, or tracheostomy?

C. Pertinent physical exam: Cardinal sign of upper airway obstruction is stridor secondary to turbulent airflow. Inspiratory stridor usually indicates partial obstruction above the vocal cords (i.e., trauma/ fractures, foreign bodies, hematomas, edema). Expiratory stridor usually indicates obstruction at or below the vocal cords. Biphasic stridor suggests partial obstruction at the level of the vocal cords. Other signs of respiratory distress may include restlessness, suprasternal retractions, and hoarseness. A hoarse voice may indicate laryngeal pathology. A muffled voice suggests supraglottic involvement, such as obstruction due to peritonsillar abscess or angioedema. Coughing or choking may be due to vocal cord paralysis, aspiration, reflux, or an anatomic abnormality (laryngeal cleft or TE fistula).

D. Work-up: Usually in a true airway emergency, there is no time for diagnostic tests until a stable airway is attained. In a less emergent setting, diagnostics include arterial blood gas, CBC, CXR, soft tissue airway films (may demonstrate supraglottic edema or subcutaneous emphysema), CT scan of the neck, and C-spine films in cases of trauma.

E. Treatment:

1. Cool humidified air helps to thin secretions and prevent crust formation. Use a face mask or face tent rather than nasal cannula if possible.

2. Oxygen per nasal cannula, face mask, face tent, or nonrebreather may be beneficial regardless of measured oxygen saturations.

3. Systemic corticosteroids may be used to acutely decrease edema from trauma, infectious, or inflammatory etiology. Dexamethasone 10 mg (Decadron) or methylprednisolone 125 mg (Solu-Medrol IV) are most commonly used as acute treatment, with Solu-Medrol having a somewhat faster onset.

4. Nebulized racemic epinephrine works quickly, acting as a topical vasoconstrictor; however, it is short-acting, and there may be a rebound effect once it dissipates. In addition, it can cause acute elevations in blood pressure which can be problematic in some patients.

5. Heliox refers to an 80%:20% helium–oxygen mixture. It relies on decreased density of helium to transport oxygen past the obstructive site. Usually used as a temporizing measure.

F. Clinical pearls:

1. Nasopharyngeal airway (nasal trumpet) is beneficial for patients emerging from general anesthesia or who have mild head trauma but normal respiratory drive. It provides support to the airway at the soft palate and base of tongue.

2. Oropharyngeal airway may treat ventilatory obstruction due to a relaxed tongue.

3. Transoral intubation is the standard for airway control. Contraindications include C-spine fractures and laryngeal or tracheal trauma. The laryngeal mask airway (LMA) is another option for emergent airway control. Use of this device is becoming more widespread and has the advantage of being placed without direct laryngoscopy.

4. Consultation is advised for possible fiberoptic intubation (in case of difficult intubation), airway distress refractory to therapeutic options, or exam of the upper airway (i.e., rule out vocal cord paralysis, neoplasm, foreign body).

5. While pulse oximetry should be monitored in a patient with airway concerns, note that saturations may stay above 95% until complete airway obstruction or respiratory exhaustion occurs. The pulmonary reserve for many patients is low and they may crash very rapidly despite initially stable pulse ox readings. *Do not let pulse oximeter readings override clinical examination of a stridulous patient.*

Tracheostomy

A. Indications/Work-up:

1. The optimal timing for a tracheostomy is controversial; however, it is accepted that earlier intervention has beneficial effects for critically ill patients. Evaluation of the patient at 7–10 days after intubation is appropriate to assess for likelihood of extubation. If long-term intubation is probable, then a tracheostomy is justified. In some patients with neuromuscular disorders or severe neurologic injury in which long-term ventilatory support is anticipated, earlier tracheostomy may be indicated.

2. Work-up for tracheostomy includes evaluation of coagulation (PT/PTT, bleeding time or PFA-100), peak airway pressures, and patient's expected prognosis.

   a. Patients on anticoagulation (including ASA) are at higher risk of both intraoperative and postoperative hemorrhage. Reverse or discontinue anticoagulation, if possible.

    b. Patients with high peak airway pressures (numbers vary, but typically over 40–45 cm H_2O) are at higher risk of ventilatory complications due to leakage of air around the tracheostomy tube at high pressures and the need for excessive cuff pressures to maintain a seal.

    c. Prognosis is a key component of discussion with the family regarding the purposes of a tracheostomy. Assistance with long ventilator weans is an appropriate indication, as is palliation of airway obstruction in end-of-life situations. A patient whose demise is imminent, however, may experience undue suffering with limited benefit from the procedure.

B. Types of tracheostomy tubes: Shiley and Portex tracheostomy tubes are plastic and come with or without cuffs. Either brand may be used initially after the surgical procedure. Typically, tracheostomy tubes are kept undisturbed for 5–7 days to allow formation of a well-healed tract. After this point, the plastic tracheostomy tubes are typically changed to a cuffless metal (Jackson) tracheostomy tube for long-term use or Shiley/Portex tubes with cuff if ventilatory support is still needed. Two types of tracheostomy may be performed: open surgical tracheostomy (performed in the operating room), or bedside percutaneous dilational tracheostomy (PDT). PDT avoids transporting a critically ill patient out of the ICU, but may be prone to complications in some patients (e.g., obese or prior neck surgery). The choice of procedure is dependent on patient characteristics, as well as the experience and preference of the surgeon.

C. Posttracheostomy care: ENT will perform the first tracheostomy tube change after 5–7 days to ensure a well-healed tract has formed. Further trach changes will typically be performed by nursing staff on the floors or by the patient/family after discharge. Frequent cleaning or changing of the inner cannula is recommended to prevent obstruction by crusting (typically at least tid). A patient with a tracheostomy should always wear a high-humidity trach collar and have suction at bedside with both a Yankauer tip and tracheal suction catheters. All patients should have a spare trach in the room similar or identical to the one they have in place. They should also have their obturator secured to the foot of the bed where it is easily accessible. The obturator is the metal or plastic inner piece that facilitates reinsertion of the trach. Nurses caring for these patients should know its location and have immediate access to it.

D. Dislodged tracheostomy tube: If the trach tube comes out, *first assess the stability of the patient.*

    1. If in respiratory distress or with stridor, call the ENT consult or Emergency Airway pager immediately for assistance. You may reinsert the tube with the aid of the obturator (which will be secured at bedside as noted above) and resecure the collar to prevent further dislodgement. *If this is not possible and the patient is decompensating, transoral endotracheal intubation is an option for most patients.* The exception is a patient with previous laryngeal surgery who may have difficult transoral airway access (or no access in the case of a patient after a total laryngectomy).

    2. If the patient is stable and comfortable, you may attempt to reinsert the trach tube as noted above. Using a small Kelly clamp to retract the skin along with a bright light source may give a better view of the tract. Occasionally, passing the trach tube over a Foley catheter or nasogastric tube will do the trick.

    3. If the patient is stridulous, talking, or breathing through the nose or mouth with the trach tube in place, it is likely in a false tract. You may feel for airflow through the trach and pass a suction catheter to confirm placement. Removing the tube and reattempting with the methods above will usually allow for correct placement. If difficulty persists, call the ENT consult pager for assistance.

E. Note: General and thoracic surgery usually perform tracheostomies when indicated for their own patients. They will manage routine questions and problems related to tracheostomies performed by their respective services.

Epistaxis

A. May be considered emergent, urgent, or routine based on volume of blood loss, hemodynamic stability, airway compromise, and whether the patient is currently bleeding. Be clear in defining the urgency of the consult when calling to elicit the appropriate rapidity of response.

B. Pertinent history: Airway status, history of facial trauma, anticoagulant medications, systemic diseases causing bleeding diatheses (e.g., hemophilia, liver disease, von Willebrand's disease, hereditary hemorrhagic telangiectasia). Use of nasal sprays, nasal cannula oxygen, and local inflammation (rhinosinusitis, allergic rhinitis, digital trauma, foreign bodies) can all contribute. Anatomic abnormalities (septal deviations or perforations) can be a cause of bleeding as well.

C. Pertinent physical exam: Ensure stable vitals. Systemic hypertension may initiate or perpetuate bleeding. Determine the source of bleeding (anterior versus posterior and right versus left naris). Identification of most anterior sites can be aided by nasal speculum and light source (headlight or mirror).

D. Work-up: Check coagulation values including PT/PTT, bleeding time or PFA-100, and hematocrit. Check blood pressure, and treat hypertension.

E. Treatment:

1. Patient should be seated completely upright to decrease risk of aspiration. For the same reason, head should be tilted slightly forward, not back.

2. Simple nasal compression for 15 minutes will stop most nosebleeds. To be effective, this must be maintained by the patient or staff without releasing pressure for the entire 15-minute period. Do not pack the nose with tissue or gauze. These will traumatize the nasal mucosa and result in further injury.

3. Control hypertension.

4. Application of topical vasoconstrictors [oxymetazoline hydrochloride 0.05% (Afrin) or phenylephrine hydrochloride 0.25%] may help to slow down bleeding.

5. If a small anterior bleeder can be visualized, it can be cauterized with judicious use of a silver nitrate stick. Never cauterize both sides of the nasal septum, as this can lead to septal perforation.

6. Remove nasal cannula O_2, which dries and irritates the nasal mucosa. Replace with humidified oxygen by face mask or tent and frequent use of nasal saline spray.

7. Nasal packing: If the above measures fail to control bleeding, nasal packing will be required. This may be performed with Vaseline strip gauze or with specifically designed nasal packs. Nasal packs should be placed by the ENT service. When calling a consult, ensure that the patient has been positioned as above and anterior nasal compression is being maintained. Set up suction at the bedside. Anterior packs can be uncomfortable, and typically require narcotics in addition to prophylactic antistaphylococcal antibiotics to prevent toxic shock syndrome. True posterior packs (Epistat) also require cardiac monitoring in an ICU or OU due to the risk of bradyarrhythmias. Packs remain in place for 3–7 days and are removed by the ENT service. Stable, reliable patients can be discharged with a pack in place and return for removal as an outpatient. If packing fails, the patient will require embolization by interventional radiology or surgical ligation of bleeding vessels.

Acute Sinusitis—Emergency

A. *This is an emergency when the infection has extended past the sinuses to involve intraorbital or intracranial structures—call a consultant immediately!*

B. Pertinent history: Duration of sinusitis symptoms, vision changes, mental status changes, duration/route of antibiotic therapy, previous sinus surgery. Predisposing factors include malnutrition, diabetes, chemotherapy, long-term corticosteroids, allergic rhinitis, immunodeficiency states, environmental exposures, and presence of nasogastric tube.

C. Pertinent physical exam: Meningeal signs and orbital signs (proptosis, chemosis, impeded extraocular movement, vision loss). These suggest extension of the infection beyond the sinus and necessitate immediate attention by an ENT consultant.

D. Work-up: Sinus CT scan, high-resolution orbital CT scan to rule out subperiosteal or orbital abscess. Head CT with IV contrast may be indicated to look for intracranial involvement.

E. Treatment:

1. IV antibiotics (broad-spectrum).

2. Copious use of saline (Ocean) nasal spray and oxymetazoline (Afrin) to aid in nasal drainage.

3. IV steroids (dexamethasone 10 mg or methylprednisolone 125 mg) to help diminish edema around orbits and reduce optic nerve damage.

4. Surgery (functional endoscopic sinus surgery or external surgical drainage) is definitive therapy to drain abscess and sinuses.

5. If optic nerve damage is imminent due to intraorbital abscess, then immediate lateral canthotomy with tendon cantholysis should be done to decrease intraocular pressure.

Vertigo

A. Vertigo emergency

1. *Important vertigo emergencies* are rare and include the following:

   a. Wallenberg's syndrome.

   b. Lateral pontomedullary syndrome.

   c. Cerebellar hemorrhage.

   d. Cerebellar infarction.

   e. Vertebrobasilar insufficiency.

2. History: Sensation and duration of dizziness, associated neurologic symptoms (headache, visual changes, unilateral weakness or paresthesias), nausea, or vomiting.

3. Physical exam: Associated neurologic findings (diplopia, dysarthria, drop attacks, vision loss, dysphagia, loss of pain/temperature sensation, loss of motor control), Horner's syndrome, nuchal rigidity, papilledema, bidirectional gaze-fixation nystagmus, absence of gaze suppression nystagmus, spontaneous upbeat or downbeat nystagmus.

4. Work-up: Neurology consultation; CT/MRI or cerebral angiogram depending on suspected etiology.

5. Treatment: Dependent on etiology, may include surgical decompression, anticoagulation, and/or supportive care.

B. Vertigo (general)

1. Common etiologies:

   a. Benign paroxysmal positional vertigo (BPPV).

   b. Ménière's disease.

   c. Vestibular neuronitis.

   d. Migraine-associated vertigo.

2. History: See Vertigo Emergency section. Differentiate true vertigo (abnormal perception of motion) from light-headedness or "off-balance." Note exacerbating factors (position changes, sudden head movement, noise), other otologic symptoms (hearing loss, otalgia, otorrhea, tinnitus), general medical history, medications. Duration and frequency of episodes are crucial to making the correct diagnosis.

3. Physical exam: Nausea and vomiting (these tend to point to peripheral cause), horizontal nystagmus, fixation suppression of nystagmus, Dix-Hallpike maneuver (BPPV).

4. Work-up: Rule out medical causes including hypotension or hypertension, cardiac arrhythmias, endocrine abnormalities.

5. Treatment: Dependent on the exact etiology (e.g., BPPV treatment requires Epley maneuver for otolith repositioning). Short-term symptomatic treatment may include the following:

   a. Compazine suppositories, 25 mg pr q6h.

   b. Meclizine (Antivert), 12.5–25 mg PO q8h prn.

   c. Diazepam (Valium), 2–10 mg PO q6h pr.

   d. For severe cases, diazepam, 5–10 mg IM or droperidol, 2.5 mg IM.

PSYCHIATRY

Key Points

A. A patient's right to refuse a psychiatric consultation:

1. Psychiatric consultation in and of itself may be stigmatizing.

2. Patients have the right to refuse consultation, *unless:*

   a. There is concern about the patient being a danger to him- or herself or others.

   b. There is concern about the patient's decision-making capacity.

3. Clinical pearl: The patient should always be told that a psychiatric consultant is coming to see him or her.

Suicidality

A. When to suspect ideation: when the patient appears sad, depressed, or anxious, when there is a significant drug or alcohol history, when there is a history of domestic abuse, when psychosis is present.

B. Before calling the consult, obtain the following information:

1. Key history: Age, gender, previous psychiatric treatment, suicide plan, presence of psychosis and command hallucinations, presence of anxiety, current meds, brief general medical history, and hospital course.

2. Key physical findings: Presence or absence of agitation, anxiety, overt psychosis.

C. Treatment:

1. Keep patient safe; get a sitter until directed otherwise by psychiatry.

2. Do not let a suicidal patient leave without clearance from psychiatry; once medical issues are resolved, the patient may require transfer to psychiatry, possibly against the patient's wishes.

D. Clinical pearls:

1. Suicidal ideation is a symptom, not a diagnosis; a full psychiatric interview is necessary to determine the cause and direct treatment.

2. Never be afraid to ask about the presence of suicidality; you will not give the patients ideas they didn't already have.

Violent Patients

A. Critical diagnostic question: Is delirium present (i.e., does the patient have a fluctuating level of consciousness with altered mental status)?

B. Before calling the consult, obtain the following information:

   1. Key history: Age, gender, onset of symptoms, level of orientation, presence of psychosis, prior psychiatric treatment, current meds, brief medical history, and hospital course.

   2. Key physical findings: Vital signs, overt psychosis, localized findings on neurologic exam.

C. Work-up: directed at identifying the cause of the delirium; may include lytes, CBC, U/A, LFTs, CSF studies.

D. Treatment:

   1. Protect the patient and staff; sedate the patient with antipsychotics (e.g., haloperidol IM in doses ranging from 0.5 mg in the frail and elderly to 5 mg in the younger and larger); use restraints if necessary.

   2. Identify and treat the cause of the delirium.

   3. Family members can help reorient delirious patients and lessen their violence. Dimly lit, quiet rooms help, as do glasses and hearing aids for those who need them.

E. Clinical pearls:

   1. Common, less obvious causes of delirium are anticholinergic medications, benzodiazepines, undertreated pain, opiates, and steroids. Offending medicines should be tapered or discontinued as much as possible.

   2. Avoid using benzodiazepines for sedation in delirious patients unless the delirium is from alcohol or sedative withdrawal, or phencyclidine intoxication.

   3. Do not put yourself in danger. Remove all possible items in the vicinity that could be used against you (e.g., stethoscope).

   4. Have security with you.

   5. Stand between the patient and an open door.

Competency

A. Definitions

   1. *Competence* is technically a legal term. Only a judge can declare someone incompetent (and appoint a guardian, for example).

2. *Decision-making capacity* refers to the ability of patients to give informed consent to medical care; psychiatrists can often assist in the assessment of capacity.

B. Competency is an emergency or urgency as the patient typically requires emergent or urgent medical care for which the patient is unable or unwilling to give consent.

C. Before calling the consult, obtain the following information:

1. Key historical information: Age, gender, proposed medical care and risks, benefits, and alternatives particular to the patient, medical history, current meds, presence of psychosis or depression, psychiatric history.

2. Key physical findings: Presence or absence of agitation, anxiety, overt psychosis.

D. Demonstration of decision-making capacity requires all *four* of the following:

1. The ability to communicate a choice.

2. Understanding of medical situation and likely outcome of no treatment.

3. Understanding of risks and benefits of treatment options.

4. Ability to manipulate information rationally and give a rational explanation for preferred treatment. *Some people add a fifth criteria which is consistency of the choice over time, but this is more controversial.*

E. Clinical pearls:

1. Many consults to psychiatry result from patients not being adequately informed of the proposed treatment's risks and benefits.

2. Presence of psychosis does not necessarily mean that a patient lacks capacity (e.g., belief that one is part of the intergalactic guard may have no bearing on understanding the risks and benefits of cardiac catheterization).

3. Capacity is decision specific; one may have capacity to take IV meds but not PO if one believes that all of the pills are sprayed with a poison.

4. Capacity is time specific. Demonstrating capacity today is no guarantee that one will be able to demonstrate capacity tomorrow should mental status fluctuate.

5. Psychiatric consultation can only help with determining if a patient lacks capacity to make a decision; the consult will not tell you who the decision-maker should be if the patient lacks capacity.

Psychosis

A. Definition: *Psychosis* is a break with reality demonstrated by hallucinations, delusions, or bizarre behavior.

B. Psychosis itself is not a psychiatric emergency. The psychiatric consult can wait until the morning. On a medical/surgical floor, psychosis is often a symptom of delirium, which can be a medical emergency.

C. Critical diagnostic question: Is the patient delirious (i.e., does the patient have a fluctuating level of consciousness with altered mental status)? If so, see the section on the violent patient for further discussion of delirium.

D. Before calling the consult, obtain the following information:

1. Key history: age, gender, previous psychiatric treatment, nature of psychosis and symptom onset, presence of anxiety, current meds, brief general medical history and hospital course, presence of suicidal or homicidal ideas, presence of command hallucinations.

2. Key physical findings: Presence or absence of agitation, anxiety, thought disorder, bizarre behavior.

E. Clinical pearls:

1. Visual hallucinations usually result from delirium or intoxication.

2. Auditory hallucinations are the most common form in psychiatric disorders.

3. Olfactory and gustatory hallucinations are usually seen in the aura of a seizure.

4. Tactile hallucinations can result from drug withdrawal.

5. Psychosis is a symptom, not a diagnosis; a full psychiatric interview is necessary to determine the cause and direct treatment.

Domestic Violence, Rape, and Psychiatric Trauma

A. Legal reporting requirements:

1. Physicians in every state are **required** to break confidentiality and report *suspected* cases of child abuse to local authorities, usually called the Division of Family Services or Child Protective Services.

2. Many states also require that suspected elder abuse be reported.

3. There are no such legal requirements for spouse abuse.

B. Rape victims should be referred to obstetrics and gynecology for collection of evidence, treatment of physical trauma, evaluation of exposure to STDs, and referred for follow-up counseling.

C. Psychiatric consultation may help with the treatment of depression, anxiety, substance abuse, posttraumatic stress disorder, and personality disorders that are all commonly found in the victims of domestic violence and rape. Perpetrators of domestic violence also frequently have many of these problems.

D. Before calling the consult, make sure the patient is willing to see a psychiatrist. Include the following information:

1. Key history: Age, gender, previous psychiatric treatment, nature of symptoms, presence of anxiety and depression, current meds, brief general medical history and hospital course, presence of suicidal or homicidal ideas.

2. Key physical findings: Presence or absence of agitation, anxiety, overt psychosis.

E. Diagnosis: Questions regarding domestic abuse should be asked as a routine part of the social history on every patient.

F. Treatment:

1. Should begin with referral to a specific domestic violence support program if one is available locally.

2. Will depend on the patient's individual symptoms.

3. Generally includes allowing the patient to tell and retell the story of the trauma in a safe, supportive environment so that the associated anxiety lessens over time.

G. Clinical pearls:

1. If in doubt, call protective services regarding child abuse for more guidance.

2. Patients rarely volunteer information on being a victim of domestic violence; the first step toward helping them is to ask.

Chemical Dependency

A. Minor alcohol withdrawal (see also Chapter 13).

1. Diagnosis:

a. Tremors, headache, nausea, sweating, and autonomic instability occurring approximately 12 hours after the last drink and lasting up to 5 days if untreated.

b. No hallucinations, seizures, or delirium.

    2. Treatment:

        a. Benzodiazepines (e.g., lorazepam 0.5–2 mg q6-8h or chlordiazepoxide 25 mg qid) given scheduled and prn to keep vital signs stable, with a gradual taper over approximately 4 days.

        b. Frequent monitoring of vital signs.

        c. Adequate hydration.

        d. Adequate replacement of electrolytes, particularly potassium and magnesium, as needed.

        e. Replacement of vitamins, especially vitamin C, folate, and thiamine.

        f. Seizure prophylaxis in those with a history of seizure.

        g. The patient should be encouraged to allow psychiatric consultation for diagnosis and treatment of a possible chemical dependency.

B. Major alcohol withdrawal (a.k.a. *rum fits* and DTs) (see also Chapter 13).

    1. This should not result in a straight psychiatric consultation. Consultation with a med-psych service or internal medicine may be appropriate, and such consultation may be emergent.

    2. Diagnosis:

        a. See the criteria under Minor alcohol withdrawal (Section A, above).

        b. Between 3 days and 2 weeks after the last drink, minor withdrawal symptoms become accompanied by hallucinations, seizures, or delirium. Autonomic instability worsens.

    3. Treatment:

        a. Same as for minor alcohol withdrawal, but monitoring of vital signs and supportive treatment are even more important; severe cases may require transfer to the ICU.

        b. Haloperidol added to the benzodiazepine can help treat hallucinosis.

        c. The patient should be encouraged to allow psychiatric consultation for diagnosis and treatment of a possible chemical dependency.

C. Cocaine and opioid withdrawal:

    1. Diagnosis:

        a. In opioid withdrawal: nausea, muscle aches, rhinorrhea, diarrhea, piloerection, and craving.

        b. In cocaine withdrawal: fatigue, agitation, increased appetite.

2. Treatment:

   a. While both conditions are unpleasant for the patient, they are rarely medically serious.

   b. Opioid withdrawal can be treated with clonidine, 0.1 mg PO tid or a methadone taper.

   c. The patient should be encouraged to allow psychiatric consultation for diagnosis and treatment of a possible chemical dependency.

D. Chemical dependency:

1. Before calling the consult, make sure the patient is willing to see a psychiatrist. Include the following information:

   a. Key history: Age, gender, previous psychiatric treatment, amount of use, route of use, withdrawal symptoms, presence of anxiety and depression, current meds, brief general medical history and hospital course, presence of suicidal or homicidal ideas, presence of psychosis.

   b. Key physical findings: Presence or absence of agitation, anxiety, overt psychosis, withdrawal signs.

2. Diagnosis: Questions regarding alcohol and substance use should be asked as a routine part of the social history on every patient.

   a. Criteria revolve around tolerance, withdrawal, and inability to control use.

   b. If two of the CAGE questions (listed here) are positive, the patient should be encouraged to allow psychiatric consultation for more definitive diagnosis. Other patients, of course, may also be appropriate for referral.

      i. Ever tried to *C*ut down?

      ii. Had others get *A*nnoyed?

      iii. Felt *G*uilty about drinking?

      iv. Had an *E*ye opener (morning drink) to avoid withdrawal?

3. Treatment:

   a. Support groups such as AA.

   b. Anticraving medication such as naltrexone, nalmefene, or ondansetron for alcoholism.

   c. Methadone maintenance (from specially licensed clinics) for severe opioid dependence.

   d. Psychotherapy aimed at relapse prevention.

   e. Treatment of comorbid depression and anxiety disorders.

4. Clinical pearls:

   a. Sedative withdrawal has the same clinical picture as alcohol withdrawal.

   b. The shorter the half-life of the benzodiazepine (e.g., alprazolam), the more likely withdrawal.

   c. Untreated DTs has a mortality of over 15%.

   d. Drug use often accompanies STDs, physical trauma, and other medical conditions.

GENERAL SURGERY

Key Points

A. Identify yourself and the patient that needs a consult, then clearly identify the question you need answered.

B. Give an indication of the urgency of the consult (i.e., STAT, a few hours, or sometime today).

C. Identify which surgical attending is requested, and then present the crucial information for the problem.

D. If important radiographs have been obtained, state their location (i.e., do not keep them in your call room).

E. Time-efficient communication is crucial. If the surgeon is abrupt, do not take personal offense, but do not use that as a personal example to follow. For example: *Hi, this is Mike. I am a medicine resident. I have an urgent consult regarding the management of a patient with a pulseless and cold foot for Dr. (Vascular Surgeon). The patient is Mr. Smith, his DOB is 5/5/45 and he is located in room 6443. He is a 62 y.o. diabetic male with CAD and severe PVD who. . . .*

Hernia

A. *A strangulated hernia is a surgical emergency—call a consult immediately!*

   1. A *reducible* hernia is one that can return through its fascial defect. An *incarcerated* hernia is one that is irreducible (impossible to push back through the fascial defect).

   2. A *strangulated* hernia is one in which the blood flow of the hernia's contents is compromised leading to necrosis of the contained structures. The signs of this are fever, leukocytosis, hypotension, erythema of the overlying skin, or extreme pain with light palpation of the hernia.

B. Pertinent information: Location and duration of the hernia, scar overlying hernia, patient's surgical history, associated symptoms and status (strangulated, incarcerated, or reducible), time of patient's last bowel movement, fever, leukocytosis, or erythema of the skin overlying the hernia. Is the patient immunocompromised?

C. Physical exam: Diagnosis of a hernia is made by examining the patient in a standing position with the patient performing Valsalva's maneuver or coughing. A mass that protrudes is a hernia until proven otherwise.

D. Treatment:

1. Attempt to reduce an incarcerated, nonstrangulated hernia that does not protrude inferior to the inguinal ligament. **Do NOT attempt to reduce a hernia that you suspect is strangulated.**

2. Place the patient supine in Trendelenburg's position and slowly apply firm, constant, circular pressure with the palm of the hand to the hernia.

   a. If the hernia reduces, then perform an abdominal examination an hour later to prove that ischemic bowel was not reduced.

   b. If the patient has abdominal pain and you suspect ischemic bowel from the hernia, call surgery urgently.

3. Most hernias require an operation if the patient can tolerate the risks of anesthesia.

4. Trusses or binders are usually not effective in the treatment of hernias.

E. Clinical pearls: Hernias are classified both by anatomy and status. Over 75% of hernias occur in the inguinal region, 10% are incisional or ventral hernias, 3% are femoral, and the rest are unusual types. The location is of less concern than the status of the hernia. Not all incarcerated hernias are strangulating. A freely reducible hernia is an elective consult that generally can wait until the morning.

Small Bowel Obstruction

A. Small bowel obstruction is an urgent consult. The most common causes are adhesions from previous abdominal operations (50%–70%), incarcerated hernias, and carcinoma. These patients always need IV fluids, a Foley catheter, and a nasogastric tube.

B. Pertinent information: The hallmarks of diagnosis are abdominal distension, nausea, vomiting, waves of abdominal pain progressing to constant pain (an ominous sign), and cessation of bowel movements.

1. Which symptoms are present? How long have they been present?
2. When was the patient's last bowel movement?
3. Is the patient febrile (and does he or she have a leukocytosis)?
4. Are there any hernias?
5. Has the patient had any previous abdominal or pelvic operations?
6. What is the output from the nasogastric tube and Foley catheter? What are the patient's vital signs and fluid status? With a persistent obstruction, hypovolemia often results due to impaired absorption, third spacing, and vomiting.
7. Does the digital rectal exam reveal impacted stool or a rectal mass?

C. Physical exam: Check for hernias in the groin, umbilicus, and all scars for incisional hernias. Are the hernias incarcerated or strangulated?

D. Diagnosis: What does the obstructive series show (do not order only a KUB), and is there colonic or rectal air? Are there air-fluid levels? Most importantly, does the radiograph demonstrate any free air? A CT scan with oral and IV contrast can be helpful to identify a transition point and subtle signs of intestinal ischemia. Be cautious of administering oral contrast to a patient with a bowel obstruction.

E. Treatment options:

1. Patients with complete bowel obstruction or peritonitis generally require prompt surgical intervention. These are often associated with strangulation of bowel.
2. Most patients with partial small bowel obstruction can be managed expectantly with nasogastric tube decompression, fluid resuscitation, serial abdominal exams, and daily abdominal plain films.

Hints for Diagnosis of an Acute Abdomen

A. An acute abdomen warrants immediate surgical intervention. These hints are not rigid rules because the diagnosis of an acute abdomen can require much judgment. The most common signs indicating an acute abdomen are peritoneal signs due to peritoneal inflammation.

. . . If there is any doubt at all, call . . .

B. Signs:

1. Rebound: This should never be tested for by pushing into the patient's abdomen and releasing. Not only is it barbaric, but also not sensitive. Instead, be gentle: pain with percussion on the anterior abdominal wall is the best test. Tapping on a patient's foot can also transmit vibrations to the abdominal cavity. Patients with an acute abdomen will not tolerate this.

2. Tussion: A patient who can cough several times without pain probably does not have peritoneal signs.

3. Laughing: A patient who laughs probably does not have peritoneal signs.

4. Sitting up for posterior chest auscultation or rolling over for a rectal examination: Most patients with peritoneal signs will not do this.

Abdominal Pain with a Pulsatile Abdominal Mass

A. *Abdominal pain with a pulsatile abdominal mass is an incredible emergency!*

B. Abdominal pain with a pulsatile abdominal mass, suggesting an AAA, is the easiest problem you will ever evaluate:

1. Call surgery for a STAT consult.

2. Type and cross the patient for 6 units of blood.

3. Ensure there is adequate IV access: at least two large bore catheters.

Ischemic Lower Extremity

A. *An ischemic extremity is an emergency—call a consult immediately!* Symptoms of acute arterial insufficiency can occur abruptly. On exam, look for the 6 P's (pain, pallor, pulselessness, paresthesias, paralysis, and poikilothermy).

B. An ischemic extremity may be due to acute events (embolic disease) or chronic disease (atherosclerosis). The acute event is an emergency because perfusion must be reestablished within 6–8 hours. Unlike patients with chronic disease, many patients with acute obstruction have not developed collateral circulation to supply the lower leg.

C. Pertinent information:

1. Suspected source: embolism (atrial fibrillation/arrhythmia, LV aneurysm, AAA, or popliteal aneurysm) or chronic disease (atherosclerosis).

2. Status of the vascular system: Has this patient had vascular surgery (if so, where does the bypass start and end?), where are the scars, and who was his or her surgeon?

D. Physical exam:

1. On exam, look for the 6 P's (pain, pallor, pulselessness, paresthesias, paralysis, and poikilothermy).

2. Status of collateral flow: Palpate or Doppler pulses in the femoral, popliteal, dorsalis pedis (DP), and posterior tibial (PT) arteries. Be able to tell the consultant if there is a temperature difference in the extremities and at what level (foot, shin, thigh, or whole leg).

3. Severity of ischemia: The most sensitive test to determine if the foot is viable is to test for proprioception of the toes. This will diminish within 5 minutes of cessation of blood flow. Next, test motor function and light touch.

E. Treatment options:

1. Most patients are started on IV heparin therapy.

2. Possible interventions include surgical bypass, surgical or interventional radiographic thrombectomy, or locally delivered intravascular thrombolytics.

Ischemic Ulcer of the Lower Extremity

A. Ischemic ulcer of the lower extremity is an elective consult.

B. Pertinent information:

1. These ulcers are commonly found on the first metatarsal head or tips of the toes and are due to a combination of unrecognized trauma, poor circulation, and infection. These are distinguished from venous stasis ulcers by location (which are usually on the lower anterior shin), vascularity (heaped up, engorged edges), and sensitivity (very painful).

2. Status of the vascular system: Has this patient had vascular surgery (if so, where does the bypass start and end?), and if so, where are the scars?

3. Have any ankle–arm indices (AAI) been performed? If not, use a Doppler and portable blood pressure cuff to do bedside AAIs. Take the SBP in the arm, then using the Doppler find a pulse in the DP or PT on the same side and blow up the BP cuff on the calf until the pulse disappears for the SBP in the foot. Divide the SBP of the foot by the SBP in the arm for the AAI on that side. Repeat on the other side.

   4. Are there any radiographs that document osteomyelitis of the underlying bone? Any exposed bone is assumed to have osteomyelitis until proven otherwise.

   5. Is the patient a diabetic? How are his blood sugars? Diabetics have elevated AAIs and can have calcified vessels. They also have poor wound healing if their diabetes is poorly controlled.

C. Pertinent physical exam: Palpate or perform a Doppler examination of the pulses in the femoral, popliteal, dorsalis pedis, and posterior tibial arteries. Look for signs of infection (e.g., erythema, pain, fluctuance, or pus discharge with palpation).

D. Treatment options:

   1. Amputation, debridement, or any procedure to increase vascular inflow in arterial disease and promote wound healing. Often these patients will need an imaging study such as a CT angio or MRA or angiogram to determine the status of the vascular supply.

   2. Leg elevation, Unna boots, or compression stockings to encourage venous drainage in venous disease.

Retroperitoneal Bleeding

A. *Retroperitoneal bleeding is an urgent consult.*

B. Retroperitoneal bleeding is most commonly seen in patients after coronary angiography and is partially due to the frequent use of anticoagulant and antiplatelet medications. The hallmark for this diagnosis is a decreasing hematocrit in a patient complaining of flank, back, or abdominal pain.

C. Pertinent information: What procedure was performed? What anticoagulants and antiplatelet agents were used, and have they been stopped? How much and how quickly has the hematocrit decreased? On the CT scan (review it yourself; do not trust the radiologist), how large is it (in centimeters)? Does it compress the urinary system, causing hydronephrosis or hydroureter, or the renal vein? These last two findings may necessitate urgent percutaneous nephrostomy tubes or surgery, respectively.

D. Pertinent physical exam: Determine the neurologic status of the patient's ipsilateral leg by having the patient perform a straight leg lift. Then test light touch is the medial and lateral upper thigh. If these senses are diminished, the patient may need urgent operative decompression of the hematoma.

E. Diagnosis: Abdominal CT scan secures the diagnosis.

F. Treatment options:

1. Variable treatment depending on situation.

2. Check CBC immediately and coags (PT/PTT/INR) and follow frequently thereafter.

3. Reverse anticoagulation with vitamin K_1 and FFP as needed. Careful coordination with cardiologists will be necessary if an intervention such as angioplasty or stenting has taken place.

4. Supportive measures (fluids, blood) and/or operative intervention.

Femoral Artery Pseudoaneurysm

A. *Emergency consultation if there is compression of the femoral nerve;* it is urgent in most other cases.

B. Pertinent information: This complication of arterial puncture occurs in the same patient population as retroperitoneal hemorrhages. What procedure was performed? What anticoagulants and antiplatelet agents were used, and have they been stopped? How large is the pseudoaneurysm by ultrasound and does it have a long, thin neck (These pseudoaneurysms are more likely to spontaneously thrombose or be amenable to ultrasound-guided compression)?

C. Physical exam: The hallmark of diagnosis is a thrill or bruit over the puncture site. Is there any evidence of emboli to the ipsilateral foot? Look at the tips of the toes and search for petechiae or new larger purple or black spots. If present, the patient may need immediate operative intervention. Is there any evidence of compression of the femoral nerve? Test motor function and light touch sensation in the leg. If absent, the patient may need immediate operative intervention.

D. Diagnosis: Ultrasound secures the diagnosis.

E. Treatment options vary from expectant management to ultrasonic compression, ultrasound-guided thrombin injection, or operative closure of the arteriotomy and evacuation of the hematoma.

Pneumothorax

A. Pneumothorax is usually an urgent consult; it is an *emergent* consult if the patient is receiving positive pressure ventilation.

B. Common symptoms include dyspnea and chest pain. Careful examination for signs of tension pneumothorax (deviation of the trachea to the opposite side, respiratory distress, and hypotension) must be performed. If there are no signs of tension pneumothorax, an upright chest x-ray should be obtained.

C. Pertinent information:

  1. What is the patient's exam and how does he or she look?

  2. Which side is affected? Is there a CXR?

  3. Is the patient on positive pressure ventilation? If so, this can be very dangerous, and you must carefully monitor the patient until tube thoracostomy is performed. Get a chest tube tray and a 28 French chest tube to the bedside. If the patient decompensates, place a 14- or 16-gauge angiocatheter in the second interspace at the midclavicular line of the affected side.

D. Treatment: Options vary as to the size and the physiologic impact of the pneumothorax:

  1. Expectant management with serial chest radiographs may suffice in a young, asymptomatic patient with a small pneumothorax who is not on positive pressure ventilation.

  2. Needle aspiration of the air collection can be performed with a three-way stopcock.

  3. Most patients may require open tube thoracostomy or percutaneous tube thoracostomy (a 16 French Thal-Quick tube).

Pleural Effusion

A. Pleural effusions are generally an elective or semi-urgent consult unless the patient is short of breath, which warrants an *emergent* consult.

B. Common symptoms include dyspnea and chest pain. Effusions can result from a wide spectrum of benign, malignant, and inflammatory conditions.

C. Pertinent information:

  1. Is the patient short of breath or having trouble breathing? Depending on the size of the effusion and the patient's pulmonary status, patients will differ in their symptomatology.

  2. Are there any CXR, chest CT, or US studies that document the effusion? Is it getting bigger?

  3. Has a thoracentesis been done? If so, what did the Gram stain/culture, pH, glucose, amylase, lactate dehydrogenase, protein levels, cell count, and cytology show of the fluid?

D. Treatment: Options vary depending on the etiology and character of the pleural effusion.

  1. Pleural effusions generally need to be drained via thoracentesis, open tube thoracostomy, or placement of a long-term catheter, such as a PleurX catheter in the acute setting.

2. Fluid should be sent off for Gram stain and culture, cytology, cell count, and biochemical analyses (pH, glucose, amylase, LDH, protein) to help discriminate between an exudative versus a transudative effusion.

3. Additional options include streptokinase for loculated effusions or pleurodesis for recurrent effusions.

Perirectal Abscess

A. Generally this is an urgent consult unless the patient is **septic**, then it is an *emergency!* Remember that there is no such thing as an unimportant abscess. It should always be evaluated by a surgeon.

B. Pertinent information: Is the patient diabetic or immunosuppressed? If so, he or she is far more likely to die or have greater morbidity from this disease. Is the patient febrile, and does he or she have a leukocytosis?

C. Physical exam:

1. Where is it (relative to the scrotum/vagina, and anus)?

2. How far does the erythema and induration extend? If the stigmata of infection extends out from the anus, the patient may have a Fournier's gangrene, which is a surgical emergency!

D. Treatment options:

1. Incision and drainage either at the bedside or in the operating room.

2. Fournier's gangrene will necessitate wide debridement in the operating room with massive irrigation of affected areas.

3. IV antibiotics.

Pressure Ulcers

A. Generally these are elective or urgent consults unless the patient is septic.

B. Pressure ulcers result from prolonged pressure to soft tissue over bony prominences. Most commonly they occur in immobile patients over the occiput, sacrum, greater trochanter, and heels.

C. Pertinent information:

1. Is the patient septic?

2. Is the patient diabetic or immunosuppressed? Has the area been irradiated in the past? What is the patient's nutritional status?

3. Is the patient immobile? What is the extent and etiology of the patient's immobility?

4. What is the duration of the ulcer?

5. What is their current wound care management?

D. Physical exam: How does it look? Where is it? How deep is it? Is there any erythema, induration, or fluctuance around it? Do you see any exposed bone?

E. Treatment options:

1. Most superficial pressure ulcers heal spontaneously when the pressure is relieved; however, this can be a lengthy process requiring over 6 months.

2. Local wound care and optimization of nutrition are key for ulcer healing. Urinary and fecal continence needs to be maintained to prevent maceration and skin breakdown.

3. Simple closure, split-thickness skin grafting, or musculocutaneous flaps are possible but often not successful unless the pressure can be removed.

Guide to Procedures

18

. . . It's just a little sting, you won't feel a thing . . .

VASCULAR ACCESS

Ultrasound-Guided Central Venous Access

The use of ultrasound guidance for the placement of central venous catheters has been shown to be superior to the landmark guided technique by improving average access time with fewer attempts, as well as by reducing rates of complications. It has been suggested that ultrasound guidance should be the method of choice for venous catheterization, especially in select populations (obese, critically ill, or history of multiple prior central venous catheters).

- *Indirect guidance* refers to assessing the vascular structures using 2D ultrasound prior to performing needle puncture and venous canalization.
- *Direct guidance* refers to using real-time ultrasound images during the needle puncture. The view can be either transverse (a cross-section of the vein) or longitudinal (visualizing the vein on its long axis). The transverse technique, which has been showed to be easier to learn by inexperienced physicians, will be described below.
- *Distinguishing veins* from arteries using ultrasound:
  1. Veins can be distinguished from arteries using ultrasound based on their easier compressibility with application of anterior-posterior pressure. Central veins tend to be larger and less circular than adjacent arteries, but this can be misleading (e.g., patients with low intra-vascular volume).
  2. The relationship of the vein to the artery can also be useful: The internal jugular is typically anterolateral to the carotid artery. The femoral vein is typically medial to the femoral artery.
  3. Doppler ultrasonography with color-flow can help identify arteries on the basis of pulsatile flow, but this can be misleading as well (e.g., patients with severe tricuspid regurgitation).

Equipment (In Addition to What Is Needed for Central Venous Access)

- A real-time 2D ultrasound machine with transducer: *Make sure it is fully charged!*
- Sterile plastic transducer sheath.
- Sterile and nonsterile ultrasound gel (sterile gel is often included with the plastic transducer sheath kit).
- A non-sterile assistant.

Procedure

1. First and foremost, track down and obtain a fully charged ultrasound machine (this may require acts of bribery in the ICU).
2. It is usually helpful to visualize the vascular structures at your access site prior to cleansing the patient. This can be done with nonsterile ultrasound gel or surgical lubricant.
   - Note the depth and caliber of the vein.
   - Evaluate for vein patency and compressibility.
   - Identify adjacent structures. (Remember: the vein is typically anterolateral to the artery for the IJ, and medial to the artery for the femoral.) *Look for an alternate site if multiple collateral vessels without a single large lumen or if a central thrombus is visualized.*
3. Cleanse and drape the patient (see central venous access section for full details).
4. Apply sterile ultrasound gel to the interior of the plastic transducer sheath. (Alternatively, your nonsterile assistant may apply nonsterile gel to the ultrasound transducer.)
5. With the aid of your nonsterile assistant, carefully lower the ultrasound transducer into the opening of the plastic sheath (ensure that the transducer does not contact the outer surface of the sheath). The sheath should be pulled by the assistant to cover the length of the transducer cord that may contact the sterile field.
6. Place sterile ultrasound gel on the patient at the selected access site.
7. Once again locate the vein at the selected entry site. Rotate the ultrasound probe to obtain the transverse view (perpendicular to the course of the vein). As for the landmark technique, you should err initially on aiming your needle away from the artery (e.g., laterally or toward the ipsilateral nipple for IJ access, and medially for femoral venous access). Before beginning, align your ultrasound view perpendicularly to your intended needle path.

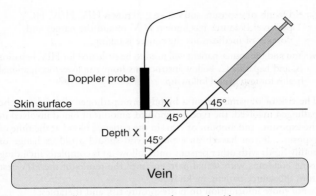

Figure 18-1 Needle insertion site using ultrasound guidance.

8. After anesthetizing the area, insert your introducer needle from the central venous access kit at a 45-degree angle to the skin at a distance away from the transducer that is approximately equal to the depth of the vein (as previously measured [see Fig. 18-1]). *When starting out, it is best to have a sterile assistant hold the ultrasound transducer allowing you to use both hands for the line placement.*

9. Once venous return is obtained the ultrasound probe may be left to the side on the sterile field (Table 18-1).

GUIDELINES FOR OCCUPATIONAL EXPOSURES

If an exposure to blood or other bodily fluids occurs:

1. *Stop what you are doing immediately!* Take a deep breath; don't panic.

2. Cleanse wound with soap and water. For mucous membrane exposures, rinse with copious amounts of water.

3. Call the hospital's exposure hotline to report the exposure and get further instructions. Each hospital has its own procedures on handling occupational exposures. When reporting an incident, you should have the following information:

   • Date and time of exposure.
   • Details of procedure being performed, amount of fluid or material exposed to, severity of exposure, type of needle used (e.g., hollow bore).

- Details of exposure source—e.g., known HIV, HBV, HCV positive? If source has known HIV, obtain the names and dosages of medications the source is taking.
4. You and the source patient will need to be evaluated for HIV, hepatitis B, and hepatitis C. Follow instructions from employee/occupational health for testing and follow-up.

The risk of transmission of a blood-borne pathogen depends on the pathogen involved, the type of exposure, amount of blood involved in the exposure, and amount of virus in the patient's blood at the time of exposure. If you have been exposed, you should avoid exchange of bodily fluids with other persons until follow-up is complete, including using condoms with sexual partners until the results of the HIV test from the source patient are known.

For more information on postexposure risk and therapies:

National Clinicians' Postexposure Hotline 1-888-448-4911 or
http://www.ucsf.edu/hivcntr/PEPline

CDC http://www.cdc.gov/ncidod/hip/Blood/exp_blood.htm

TABLE 18-1   ALL YOU REALLY NEED TO KNOW ABOUT VASCULAR ACCESS

Type	Description	Common Uses	Duration of Use
Triple-lumen catheter	Three separate lumens. Placed via the Seldinger technique usually at the bedside. Subclavian or internal jugular veins preferred, femoral vein can be used.	When peripheral access is exhausted and in emergency situations. Blood may be drawn from the catheter.	Short-term use. Replace femoral lines more frequently (~3 days).
Hickman catheter	Surgically placed (single or multilumen). Subcutaneously tunneled. Dacron cuff at the skin entry site. Located in subclavian vein (tip is located near the right atrium).	Long-term intravenous medications and/or fluids. Blood may be drawn from the catheter.	Long-term use. May be left in place indefinitely as long as functioning properly.
Hohn catheter	Single- or double-lumen Silastic catheters. Placed via Seldinger technique by interventional radiology or surgery *without* a subcutaneous tunnel.	Placed when peripheral access is exhausted. Administration of medications and fluids (when double-lumen). Blood may be drawn from the catheter.	Intermediate-term use (up to 6 weeks).

(Continued)

191

TABLE 18-1	ALL YOU REALLY NEED TO KNOW ABOUT VASCULAR ACCESS *(Continued)*		
Type	**Description**	**Common Uses**	**Duration of Use**
Implanted venous access device (Port-A-Cath)	Antimicrobial cuff at the skin insertion site. Located in subclavian or internal jugular veins. Placed subcutaneously by a surgeon or interventional radiology. Single or double lumen. Specialized right-angle needle is required to access the portal chamber. Located in subclavian vein; tip is located near the right atrium.	Long-term intravenous medications and/or fluids, especially chemotherapy. Blood may be drawn from the catheter.	Intended for indefinite use.
Tunneled cuffed catheters (ASH, Duraflow, Tesio, etc.)	Dual lumen sialastic catheters. Placed by intervential radiology. Can be placed in the internal jugular vein or subclavian vein.	Used for hemodialysis. Do not use catheter for any other reason without checking with nephrologist.	Intermediate-term use to allow graft or fistula maturation, if patients refuse permanent access, or if graft or fistula is contraindicated.

Midline catheter	*Kink proof* material. Peripherally placed by trained nursing personnel. Located in antecubital vein. Consider the possibility of midline catheter placement early before potential peripheral vessels are damaged.	Intermediate-term intravenous medications are planned (e.g., a several-week course of antibiotics). Not intended for TPN or chemotherapy. Blood drawing is discouraged (causes fibrin deposition at the tip and eventual catheter failure). Intended for indefinite use.	Intermediate-term use (1–6 weeks). Heparin flushing should be performed when the catheter is not being used for therapy at least twice a day.
PICC	17-inch Silastic catheter placed by trained nursing personnel. Interventional radiology can place PICC lines under fluoroscopy if necessary. Located in basilic, cephalic, or median cubital vein.	Long-term intravenous medications are planned. TPN and irritant medications provided the tip is in the superior vena cava. Blood may be drawn from the catheter.	Long-term use. May be left in place indefinitely as long as functioning properly.

Critical Care Notes

19

. . . Survival of the fittest . . .

KEYS TO INTENSIVE CARE UNIT SURVIVAL

. . . Always come back to the basics: Air goes in and out. Blood goes round and round. Oxygen is good . . .

- Transfer notes (see Chapter 6) with key details of the patient's past medical history and course are always helpful. The primary physician, receiving physician, and the patient's family members should be notified. Note any details or special situations that need attention and/or follow up.

- Admitting a patient to an intensive care unit can be intimidating, but keep in mind the ABCs (airway, breathing, circulation) and focus on stabilizing the patient.

- Be nice to the nurses, respiratory therapists, and other ancillary staff during your stay. They can often make useful suggestions, catch things you miss, and be immensely helpful to you in critical situations. They can be the difference between an enjoyable or miserable experience.

- Ask (and keep asking) if you have questions or problems. Mistakes from inexperience in critically ill patients can have catastrophic consequences.

- Always treat the patient, not the numbers.

- It's always a good idea to make rounds on patients and follow up on labs several times a day even if things seem stable.

- Daily ICU notes should include ventilator settings, I/O's, pulmonary artery catheter measurements, medications and drips (antibiotics, sedatives, pressors), nutritional status, and documentation of every indwelling catheter or tube.

- References to have nearby at all times:
  - Winshall JS, Lederman RJ. *Tarascon Internal Medicine and Critical Care Pocketbook*, 4th ed. Tarascon Publishing, 2006.
  - Marino PL, Sutin KM. *The ICU Book*, 3rd ed. Baltimore: Lippincott Williams & Wilkins, 2006.

- Kollef MH, Micek ST. Critical Care. In *Washington Manual of Medical Therapeutics*, 32nd ed. Philadelphia: Lippincott Williams & Wilkins, 2007.

VENTILATORS

. . . Breathe in, breathe out . . .

Suggestions for Initial Ventilator Settings

Basic Settings
- Mode
  - CMV/AC: Guarantees set tidal volume; often best to start with this.
  - SIMV + PSV: Choreographed breaths at preselected rate; allows spontaneous breaths.
  - PCV: Pressure controlled ventilation; can't guarantee the tidal volume if lung compliance decreases.
- Tidal volume: 10–12 mL/kg versus 5–7 mL/kg in low tidal volume, lung protective ventilation.
- Rate: 10–15 breaths/minute.
- FIO_2: 1.0, then titrate down (patients should never be ventilated on 100% O_2 >24 hours unless absolutely necessary).
- PEEP: 0–5 cm H_2O (careful with auto-PEEP).

Advanced Settings
(Ask for help before you change these)
- Inspiratory flow: 50–60 L/min. With COPD may want as high as 100 L/min.
- I:E ratio: 1:2. This must be set individually with PCV.
- Peak and plateau pressures: Attempt to keep peak pressure <45 cm H_2O and plateau pressure <35cm H_2O.

Ventilator Adjustments

- A PO_2 of 60 mm Hg or greater is usually the goal. Oxygenation is most affected by mean air pressure. Adjustments to FIO_2 and PEEP can help increase oxygenation. Remember that the oxygen saturations tell you nothing about the PO_2.
- CO_2 is regulated by ventilation. Increasing the respiratory rate or tidal volume blows off more CO_2.
- See Table 19-1 for suggested adjustments.

TABLE 19-1	SUGGESTIONS FOR VENTILATOR MANAGEMENT BASED ON P_{CO_2} AND P_{O_2}*	
	P_{CO_2}	P_{O_2}
High	↑ Minute volume ↑ Tidal volume ↑ Respiratory rate	Decrease F_{IO_2}
Low	↓ Minute volume ↓ Tidal volume ↓ Respiratory rate	PEEP ± Increased F_{IO_2} (in cases of diffusion block, increase F_{IO_2})

*Individualize for every patient.

General "Ballpark" Change Guidelines

- Desired P_{O_2} >60 mm Hg. Use this simple ratio to calculate the required F_{IO_2} (defined as X):

$$\text{Current } P_{O_2}/\text{Desired } P_{O_2} = \text{Current } F_{IO_2} (\%)/X (\%)$$

$$(\text{e.g., if } P_{O_2} \text{ is 150 on 100\% } O_2 \ldots)$$

$$150/60 = 100/X = 40\%$$

The F_{IO_2} can be reduced to 0.4 and this should maintain a P_{O_2} of 60.

- Desired P_{CO_2}. Another simple formula:

$$P_{CO_2} (\text{current rate}) = \text{desired } P_{CO_2} (X)$$

$$X = \text{New rate to set to obtain the desired } P_{CO_2}$$

Worsening Oxygenation

The knee-jerk impulse is to turn up the F_{IO_2}. Don't panic, approach the problem in a stepwise manner:

- Is there a ventilator problem?
  - Is the ET tube in the correct position or has it migrated? Check with the nurse on the marking of the ET tube and the most recent x-ray.
  - Is there a cuff leak or kink in the ET tube? Have respiratory therapy check this.

- Recheck the ventilator settings. Have there been inadvertent changes?
- Is there an obstruction in the ET tube (e.g., mucous plug)? Suction now.
- Is it a patient-related problem (e.g., biting, agitation)? Sedation may be needed.
- Always consider pneumothorax. Listen on both sides and consider a CXR.
- Is the underlying problem worsening? Is the patient fluid overloaded or is there bronchospasm? Is a PE a possibility? Has ventilator-associated pneumonia developed?
- Is the patient oversedated? Do you need to rethink the mode of ventilation? Check the PEEP level at end-expiration. Hypoxemia can be from a loss of PEEP.

Weaning Parameters

The method of weaning is not as relevant as knowing the appropriate time to wean. (See Table 19-2.)

TABLE 19-2	GUIDELINES FOR ASSESSING WITHDRAWAL OF MECHANICAL VENTILATION

Patient's mental status: awake, alert, cooperative
Po_2 >60 mm Hg with an Fio_2 <0.5
PEEP ≤5 cm H_2O
Pco_2 and pH acceptable
Spontaneous tidal volume >5 mL/kg
Vital capacity >10 mL/kg
Minute ventilation <10 L/min
Maximum voluntary ventilation double of minute ventilation
Maximum negative inspiratory pressure ≥25 cm H_2O
Respiratory rate <30 breaths/min
Static compliance >30 mL/cm H_2O
Rapid shallow breathing index <100*
Stable vital signs following a 1 to 2 hour spontaneous breathing trial

*Rapid shallow breathing index = Respiratory rate/tidal volume in liters.

From Kollef MH, Micek ST. Critical Care. in Cooper DH (Ed). *Washington Manual of Medical Therapeutics*, 32nd ed. Lippincott Williams & Wilkins, 2007.

ICU SEDATION

. . . Sleep tight . . . pleasant dreams . . .

- Ventilated patients generally require sedation. This is usually achieved through continuous IV infusion of sedatives. See Table 19-3.
- Achieve the desired level of sedation with boluses before starting infusion. Level of sedation is commonly measured by the modified Ramsey scale:

Level	Patient Response
1	Patient anxious, agitated, or restless
2	Patient cooperative, oriented, and tranquil
3	Patient asleep, responds to commands only
4	Patient asleep, responds to gentle shaking
5	Patient asleep, does not respond to auditory stimulus, responds to noxious stimulus
6	Patient has no response to firm nailbed pressure or other noxious stimuli

- If the patient becomes agitated, rebolus to desired level of sedation and then make small increments in the drip rate.
- Titrate to minimum effective dose and reassess the need for continuous sedation daily.
- Consider adding paralytics for patients with very poor oxygenation or if agitation persists despite adequate sedation, causing difficulty with ventilation. Make sure the patient is adequately sedated before adding paralytics!

CARDIAC PARAMETERS

. . . Don't go breaking my heart . . .

- Normal cardiac output
  - 5 ± 1 L/min
- Normal cardiac index
  - 3 ± 0.54 min/m^2
- Normal filling pressures
  - Right atrial pressure 0–8 mm Hg
  - Right ventricular pressure 5–30/0–8 mm Hg

TABLE 19-3 DRUGS FOR ICU SEDATION AND PARALYSIS

	Bolus Dosing			Continuous Infusion		
Drug	**Bolus Dosing**	**Onset (Single Dose)**	**Duration (Single Dose)**	**Dilution**	**Maintenance**	**Comments**
Fentanyl	50–100 µg	1–2 min	30–60 min	2500 µg/ 50mL	50–100 µg/hr, ↑ in 50 µg/hr increments to max 500 µg/hr	Possible bradycardia with bolus doses. Effects prolonged in renal and hepatic failure.
Morphine	10–15 mg	5–10 min	3–4 hr	100 mg/ 100 mL	1–4 mg/hr, ↑ by 2–5 mg/hr to max 50 mg/hr	Possible hypotension. Effects prolonged in renal and hepatic failure.
Lorazepam	2–4 mg	20–40 min	3–6 hr	40 mg/ 40 mL	0.5 mg/hr, ↑ by 0.25 mg/hr,to max 4 mg/hr	Effects prolonged in renal and hepatic failure.
Midazolam	1–5 mg	1–4 min	30–60 min	50 mg/ 50 mL	1 mg/hr, ↑ by 1 mg/hr to max 10 mg/hr	Possible hypotension with bolus. Effects prolonged in renal and hepatic failure.

(Continued)

TABLE 19-3 DRUGS FOR ICU SEDATION AND PARALYSIS (*Continued*)

Drug	Bolus Dosing			Continuous Infusion		
	Bolus Dosing	Onset (Single Dose)	Duration (Single Dose)	Dilution	Maintenance	Comments
Propofol	0.3 mg/kg (optional)	1–2 min	30 min	1,000 mg/ 100 mL	25–50 µg/kg/ min; ↑ by 10 µg/ kg/min to max 100 µg/kg/min	Possible hypotension, bradycardia.
Dexmedetomidine	1 µg/kg over 10 min	10 min	30 min	200 µ/ 100 mL	0.2–0.7 µg/ kg/hr, ↑ by 0.1 µg/kg/hr	Possible hypotension, bradycardia. Do not use for <24 hours.

Adapted from *Barnes-Jewish Hospital Guidelines for ICU Sedation and Therapeutic Paralysis.* Barnes-Jewish Hospital Department of Pharmacy. St. Louis: Washington University Medical Center, 2004.

- Pulmonary artery pressure 15–30/3–12 mm Hg
- Pulmonary wedge pressure 3–12 mm Hg

SHOCK

. . . We're not talking about the electrical kind . . .

Hemodynamic Profiles Associated with Shock

	CVP	CI/CO	SVR	SvO$_2$	PCWP
Hypovolemic (e.g., hemorrhage)	↓	↓	↑	↓	↓
Cardiogenic (e.g., MI, tamponade)	↑	↓	↑	↓	↑
Distributive (e.g., septic)	↓	↑	↓	N-↑	N-↓

CVP = central venous pressure; CI = cardiac index; CO = cardiac output; SVR = systemic vascular resistance; SvO$_2$ = mixed venous oxygen saturation; PCWP = pulmonary capillary wedge pressure; N = normal.

Treatment of Shock

- Determine the type of shock you are dealing with.
- Fluid resuscitation is vital, especially for hypovolemic shock. Crystalloids (normal saline or Lactated Ringer's) should be started immediately. For hemorrhagic shock, blood products should be administered.
- Use of vasopressors and inotropes can be helpful. These are generally titrated to a mean arterial pressure of ≥60 mm Hg. Afterload reduction may be helpful in cardiogenic shock. *See Drips section below for dosages.*

DRIPS

. . . And we're not talking about from your faucet . . .

See Table 19-4 for common drips used in the ICU.

TABLE 19-4   COMMON DRIPS USED IN THE ICU

	Receptor Activity	Dosage	Comments
Vasopressors			
Dopamine	α, β, dopamine	2–3 μg/kg/min for renal and splanchnic 4–8 μg/kg/min for increase in cardiac contractility (β) >10 μg/kg/min for vasoconstriction (α)	Dose-dependent receptor activation.
Epinephrine	α β	Start at 1–4 μg/min, titrate to MAP ≥60	Drug of choice for anaphylactic shock. Potent vasoconstrictor.
Norepinephrine	α β	Start at 2 μg/min, titrate to MAP ≥60	Vasoconstrictor.
Vasopressin	V1a, V1b, V2	0.04 U/minute	Has inotropic and chronotropic properties, causes reflex peripheral vasodilation.
Dobutamine	α, β	Start at 3 μg/kg/min, titrate ≤20 μg/kg/min	Inotrope, direct peripheral vasodilator.
Milrinone	PDE III inhibitor	0.375–0.75 μg/kg/min	
Vasodilators/Afterload reducers			
Nitroglycerin	Stimulates cGMP production resulting in vascular smooth muscle relaxation	Start at 5–10 μg/kg/min, titrate 10–20 μg/kg/min every 5 min until desired effect	At high doses, reflex tachycardia can occur, patients can develop tolerance to medication.
Nitroprusside	Direct peripheral vasodilator	Start at 0.25 μg/kg/min, maximum 10 μg/kg/min	Check sodium thiocyanate level with prolonged use; do not use in renal failure.

SUGGESTIONS FOR PROPHYLAXIS

. . . An ounce of prevention is worth a pound of cure . . .

- DVT: see DVT prophylaxis section, Chapter 8.
- GI: see GI prophylaxis section, Chapter 8.
- Decubitus ulcers: Turn patient several times a day, vigilant skin care, egg-crate mattress or Kin-Air bed, and adequate nutrition.
- Deconditioning: Physical therapy and nutritional support.
- Aspiration precautions: Elevate head of the bed and frequent suctioning (especially around the cuff of ET tube).
- Seizure or fall precautions: As appropriate.
- Infection: Maintain oral hygiene, keep track of lines (IV, NG tube, feeding tubes) and change per protocol, and target or discontinue antibiotic therapy to avoid resistance and *C. difficile* colitis.
- Follow isolation (respiratory or contact) precautions at all times, and wash your hands!

TOTAL PARENTERAL NUTRITION (TPN)

. . . A viable GI tract is a terrible thing to waste . . .

- Consider this option if the GI tract is unusable for at least 7 days. Sterile vascular access is needed.
- Administer through the brown port of the triple lumen catheter. Reserve this port if you think initiating TPN is a possibility—cannot be used if it has been used previously.
- For initial orders and questions, a **nutritional support consult** will be valuable for information, advice, other options, and help with calculating projected nutritional needs.
- TPN orders must be written daily and received by a certain time— make sure this is done before signing out.
- Monitor vital signs, daily weight, I/Os, Accu-Cheks, and routine labs (CBC, electrolytes, BUN, SMA–9, Mg) frequently. Monitor triglycerides and hepatic function at least once a week.
- May add H_2 blockers, steroids, insulin, and vitamin K to TPN if so desired.
- If TPN must be stopped, monitor blood sugar and administer IV fluids (e.g., D_{10}) at the same rate.

Final Touches

20

. . . Words to the wise and sleep deprived . . .

1. When in doubt, ask and ask again. Call someone (wake up someone if you need to), preferably someone who knows more than you do.

2. When in doubt, it's always better (albeit more painful) to go see the patient.

3. The right thing to do usually involves less sleep.

4. Walk if you don't need to run. Sit down if you don't need to stand. Lie down if there's a bed nearby. Answer all of nature's calls.

5. Take primary responsibility for your patients—you are their doctor.

6. Listen to your patients. They'll usually tell you what you need to know.

7. Resist the temptation to discuss patient care in public areas; no good can come of it.

8. A healthy amount of companion and compulsion makes it difficult to harm patients.

9. See one, do one, teach one. You'll be expected to assume more teaching responsibilities as time goes on. Start developing your own teaching style and discuss expectations clearly with all learners.

10. Help out your colleagues. If you finish your work early, check with other members of your team or the cross-covering intern to see if they need anything; they can return the favor when you need it most.

11. Before going home for the day, make sure your patients are tucked in, and check out with your resident. A complete sign-out is vital—make sure to include any information (studies, consults, procedures) that may be needed to make major therapeutic decisions. Be sure to leave a pager number in case complicated issues arise that need your expertise about the patient.

12. Worthy goals for internship include learning to distinguish the life-threatening issues from the acute ones from the stable ones; mastering the interpretation and proper usage of diagnostic tests; learning procedural skills; refining the ability to ask specific questions for every consult you request.

13. Fear and anxiety are normal. Take a deep breath and plunge in—there are people around to help you.

14. There is no magic spell on the last day of internship that will turn you into a resident. Trust that if you do and learn the right things during internship, you will be prepared to rise to the challenges of residency.

15. Residency, too, shall prn.

PATIENT DATA TRACKING FORM

Name		
DOB		Age
Admitted		Discharged
Allergies		

HPI
PMH/PSH
Admission Meds
SH   FH
ROS
Admission

T		P		R		BP
O_2				Wt		Ht

MCV=
RDW=

C_A		T bili		PTT			
Mg		D bili		PT			
Phos		AST		INR			
TP		ALT		Amylase			
Alb		Alk Ph		Lipase			

Previous Labs:

EKG   CXR
Admission: Admission:
Previous: Previous:
Previous Studies:

Problems:

Brief Course:

ADMISSION	DISCHARGE
☐ Old data	☐ Placement
☐ Old records	
☐ DDx	☐ Home care
☐ Admit orders	
☐ Interview	☐ D/C orders
☐ H&P	
☐ Schedule tests	☐ Transport
☐ Read	
☐ DVT Proph	

Date							
Overnight Complaints							
	CP		SOB		CP		SOB	
	N/V		Abd		N/V		Abd	
	Urine		Ap/wt		Urine		Ap/wt	
	Fatigue		BM		Fatigue		BM	
	HA		Vis		HA		Vis	
	Aud				Aud			
Meds							
Relevant Tests							
T (T$_{max}$)							
P							
R							
BP							
SaO2							
I/O							
Accu							
Physical Exam							

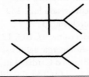 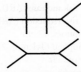

Other Labs					

Tasks	□ Pre-round
	  □ Notes in chart
	  □ Vitals
	  □ Meds
	  □ Labs
	  □ Micro
	□ Note
	□ Order tests
	□ AM Labs
		□ Change meds
		□ Call consults
		□ Read consults
		□ Talk with other team members
		□ Test Results
		□ Chat with pt and loved ones
			□ Pre-round
			  □ Notes in chart
			  □ Vitals
			  □ Meds
			  □ Labs
			  □ Micro
			□ Note
			□ Order tests
			□ AM Labs
				□ Change meds
				□ Call consults
				□ Read consults
				□ Talk with other team members
				□ Test Results
				□ Chat with pt and loved ones	

A/P					

Index

$F_iO_2 = 20\%$

N.C. $\times 4 + 20 = F_iO_2$

$(6 L\ N.C.) \times 4 + 20 \Rightarrow$ ~~44%~~ 44%

<u>VM</u> (venti mask) $\Rightarrow$ if mouth breathing

24%; 28%, 31%, 35%, 40%

<u>FM</u> (face mask)

$\Rightarrow > 55\%$

<u>NRB</u> (non rebreather)   arterial oxygen partial pressure

$\Rightarrow > 90\%$ $(P_aO_2 \Rightarrow 5 \times F_iO_2)$

$pH\ |\ CO_2\ |\ P_aO_2\ |\ HCO_3^-\ |$ Sat

$\qquad\quad$ CO (cardiac output
$\qquad\qquad\qquad\qquad$ arterial O_2
$\qquad\qquad\qquad\qquad\qquad$ content

$DO_2 = Q \times C_aO_2 \times 10$

O_2 delivery
$\quad$ equation

$\qquad\qquad (1.34 \times [Hb] \times S_aO_2) + (0.031 \times P_aO_2)$

$\qquad\qquad\qquad$ pulse ox. $\rightarrow O_2$ in Plasma
$\qquad\qquad\qquad\qquad\qquad\qquad\qquad\qquad\qquad \rightarrow$ help calc.
$\qquad$ carrying $\qquad\qquad$ A-a gradient
$\qquad$ capacity SpO_2 $\qquad\qquad\qquad$ $\Rightarrow$ constant! important in
$\qquad\qquad\qquad\qquad\qquad$ (Raynauds; cold; MetHb; CO p ??.) hypoxemia

O_2 on Hb

$\qquad\qquad$ alveolus

$Q \rightarrow$

$\begin{array}{l} V/CO \\ ;PE \\ Q \end{array}$ $\dfrac{V\uparrow}{Q\downarrow} \Rightarrow$ vent.wt > 1
                            no oxygen
$\qquad$ blood $\uparrow$ dead space

$\dfrac{V\downarrow}{Q\uparrow} \Rightarrow \downarrow < 1$
$\qquad \Rightarrow$ asthma, COPD; interstitial edema